"A remarkable book as it exposes the complex destinies of refugees through encounters with individuals and groups. The author uses herself as a tool in understanding the unique mental and social situations of the 'Refugee People' in a way that makes the reader understand better what it means to be a human being under such extreme circumstances. In this way, they come alive in the reader's mind and hopefully also contribute to the better of an important group of our fellow human beings."

Sverre Varvin, *Professor Emeritus, OsloMet—Oslo Metropolitan University, Training Analyst Norwegian Psychoanalytic Society*

"*A Psychoanalytic Approach to Refugee Mental Health: Safe Harbor* is a ground-breaking exploration that offers profound insights into human resilience, trauma, and healing. By illuminating the complex psychological landscapes of refugees and their caregivers, Chrysi Giannoulaki provides a compassionate, nuanced approach to understanding displacement, violence, and the restoration of human connection. The book is a vital contribution to our understanding of trauma and the transformative potential of psychoanalytic practice."

Danielle Knafo, *author of Living with Terror, Working with Trauma: A Clinician's Handbook*

"This book addresses a crucial current problem: the movement of refugee populations whose tragic adversity in integrating into a foreign society is exacerbated by a lack of understanding of their mental reality. Dr Chrysi Giannoulaki, with her empathy and scientific systematicity, highlights the difficulties of communicating with people from different cultural traditions. Reading this book is particularly interesting and valuable for those involved in helping refugees. It is about expanding the possibilities when dealing with a permanent feature of contemporary global political and cultural development."

Dr Nikolaos Tzavaras, *Honorary President of the Hellenic Psychiatric Association, Training Analyst of the Hellenic Psychoanalytic Society*

A Psychoanalytic Approach to Refugee Mental Health

A Psychoanalytic Approach to Refugee Mental Health reflects on psychoanalytic work with vulnerable people during the refugee crisis.

Chrysi Giannoulaki describes her work as a supervisor of groups of caregivers dealing with the mental health of refugees and occasionally as a psychiatrist of refugees in Moria, Lesvos, and in Athens. The book explores work with complex refugee cases that involve major economic, political, and social issues, with victims of sexual violence, and with unaccompanied minors. Exploring the potential of psychoanalytic theory of trauma and psychosis, clinical psychoanalytic thinking to foster integration, and tolerance of the extremely traumatized individual within networks of social relations, the book acts protectively against moments of xenophobia and polarization.

A Psychoanalytic Approach to Refugee Mental Health will be essential reading for psychoanalytically informed mental health professionals, especially those working with refugees, asylum seekers, and vulnerable patients.

Chrysi Giannoulaki is a psychiatrist and a training analyst of the Hellenic Psychoanalytic Society. She is a full member of the Psychiatry and Art Section of the Hellenic Psychiatric Association, whose actions aim to enhance awareness of racism and xenophobia. Chrysi has been working with refugees since 2016.

IPA in the Community
Series Editor: Harvey Schwartz

Applying Psychoanalysis in Medical Care
Edited by Harvey Schwartz

Trauma, Flight and Migration
Psychoanalytic Perspectives
Edited by Vivienne Elton, Marianne Leuzinger-Bohleber, Gertraud Schlesinger-Kipp and Vivian B Pender

Psychoanalytic Work in East Africa
Barbara Saegesser

Exploring Eating Disorders Through Psychoanalysis
Unravelling the Psyche
Humberto Lorenzo Persano

A Psychoanalytic Approach to Refugee Mental Health
Safe Harbor
Chrysi Giannoulaki

For more information about this series, please visit: www.routledge.com/IPA-in-the-Community/book-series/IPAC

A Psychoanalytic Approach to Refugee Mental Health

Safe Harbor

Chrysi Giannoulaki

Routledge
Taylor & Francis Group

LONDON AND NEW YORK

Designed cover image: Getty | Abstract Aerial Art

First published 2026
by Routledge
4 Park Square, Milton Park, Abingdon, Oxon OX14 4RN

and by Routledge
605 Third Avenue, New York, NY 10158

Routledge is an imprint of the Taylor & Francis Group, an informa business

British Library Cataloguing-in-Publication Data
A catalogue record for this book is available from the British Library

ISBN: 978-1-041-07138-9 (hbk)
ISBN: 978-1-041-07137-2 (pbk)
ISBN: 978-1-003-63902-2 (ebk)

DOI: 10.4324/9781003639022

Typeset in Palatino
by Deanta Global Publishing Services, Chennai, India

To the community of refugees from Sirince to the small village of Taxiarchis in Evia, Greece, to their nostalgic narratives of their hometown, to their songs and way of life they brought with them, to their fight to survive. From them to all the refugees.

Contents

Preface

Let us go back to 2015 when the "number of sea arrivals in Greece hits the half million mark" and when "UNHCR warns of continued chaos unless the reception process in the Aegean islands is strengthened," as Tim Gaynor writes for UNHCR (20. Oct 2015).

The vast number of refugee arrivals flooded the islands and reached the waterfront of ships in Piraeus. When I went to provide food, clothes, and stationery for the children as requested by humanitarian organizations at the time, I was deeply distraught. I began to wonder how I could contribute to the relief of even one refugee or to the empowerment of even one of those most directly involved in the care of refugees. In addition, I felt a burning desire to step outside the usual practice at my office and the Hellenic Psychoanalytic Association and offer what I have learned and acquired from previous generations of psychoanalysts to the community.

I believe that the complexity of the refugee issue, which is moral, economical, legal, political, and essentially global, can better be acknowledged with the contribution of psychoanalytic thought. This book is the fruit of my work in the refugee field over the past eight years through different organizations in Lesvos and Athens.

The publication of the book in the IPA in the Community series materializes my desire to contribute to the strengthening of the bonds between psychoanalysis and the community, continuing the efforts of colleagues like the authors of the texts contained in the book *Trauma, Flight and Migration: Psychoanalytic Perspectives* (Leuzinger-Bohleber et al. 1, 2023), whom I sincerely thank for the inspiration their work is for me.

Acknowledgments

I would like to start with the Medecins Du Monde and, more specifically, with Dr Nikitas Kanakis and Professor Nikos Tzavaras, who invited me to go to Moria, Lesvos, to support the team of professionals working with refugees. This collaboration allowed me to become involved with the refugees and their caregivers and continue in Athens. I would also like to thank EPAPSY and Médecins Sans Frontières for cooperating in the refugee field. In addition, I would like to thank all the caregivers and members of the supervision groups who, through the continuous sharing of their experiences, stimulated the desire to persist in the refugee field.

Without the invitation from Vivienne Elton, Marianne Leuzinger-Bohleber, Gertraud Schlesinger-Kipp, and Vivian B. Pender to participate in the collective book *Trauma, Flight, and Migration*, it would not have occurred to me to publish my experiences and thoughts in English. Professor Anna Christopoulou, with whom we cowrote one chapter of the above book, was also a person with whom the constant exchange of views and information she offered me on the international scene of psychoanalytic discussions has been a valuable support over the last 20 years.

Mr Ioannis Vartzopoulos, editor of the Greek psychoanalytic journal *Oedipus* and *Oedipus Annual*, assigned me articles about refugees as a center of interest. This provided me with a safe space to present my thoughts, ultimately leading to the formation of this book.

The trust of the editor Harvey Schwartz and the patience of Susannah Frearson, until I ventured to compile the work of about eight years into a book, have been of great help to me, and I would like to express my gratitude to them.

I am also indebted to the psychoanalysts Françoise Davoine and Jean-Max Gaudilliere for the valuable journey we have traveled together and the friendship with which they honored me. The books we dealt with during our visits to Paris have accompanied me on my journey throughout the intervening years. Their advice has remained alive in me, as seen in this book, and has oriented me as a beacon through various difficult moments of my journey. It is one of the reasons I did not feel alone in once-lonely circumstances.

Another reason why I did not feel alone was the warm communication and exchange of thoughts with Petros Hartokollis and Mr Nikos Kouretas, whose professional migration trip to the United States was an additional reason for my visits to the psychoanalytic community of New York, where I met many friends. Amid this, the friendship of Rita Clark and her husband Julian has been important to me.

I will return to Professor Nikos Tzavaras, whose meeting with him when I was still a resident psychiatrist paved the way for me to understand transference and countertransference with psychotic patients with an approach based beyond the work of Sigmund Freud on the work of Karl Jaspers and philosophers such as Friedrich Nietzsche. I feel exceptionally fortunate that his erudition and scientific excellence enriched my perspective on human nature early in my career.

I have no words to express my gratitude to Ms. Natasha Hassiotis for her emotional and practical support, which made completing this book possible. Her knowledge of English and psychoanalysis was a sine qua non condition for the last and important stop of the journey.

Finally, I owe much to my husband, Nikos Karapanagos, and my children, George and Anastasia, for their patience as they share the time I spend writing, even on vacation.

Introduction

The opening verses of the *Odyssey* outline the concept of the search for the father by the son and the mediation of the son at the beginning of the father's homecoming with the intervention of Athena, who represents the divine element. Telemachus is pushed on a journey that is *a quest for the father* in the cities of Pylos and Sparta. His journey is his father's journey in miniature. Telemachus travels to find his father. Odysseus travels to return to his homeland. The position of man as a link between generations is thus highlighted as of paramount importance. We are all nostalgic for a journey where we will meet our ancestors and settle our accounts with them. Are we the ones through whom part of their journey will be "put into words"? Will our journey be a legacy for future generations to carry on?

However, the journey of Odysseus and his son Telemachus follows another war epic, *the Iliad*, which begins with the conflict between King Agamemnon and the great warrior Achilles. The two men belong to different generations (another father–son-like relationship) and quarrel over a woman named Briseis. The clash of generations and the great anger of Achilles toward the leader of the Achaeans, Agamemnon, was the beginning of the Homeric epics. Before leaving Greece for Troy, Agamemnon promised his daughter Iphigenia that he would give her Achilles as her husband to lure her to her sacrifice.

At the Delphi conference on *The Father*, Claudio Laks Eizirik said that in the field of mythology, it is recorded in different traditions that patriarchal societies, to exist and expand, rely on dysfunctional father–son relationships, which prove that the process of separation and differentiation from a frightening giant paternal figure is carried out relentlessly and extremely (Bazaridis 2023, 41). War (is the) father of all, as the dark philosopher Heraclitus claimed. At the beginning of my journey toward writing this book, I first met war.

Meeting War – Madness and Trauma

As far back as 1998, I attended a talk on *Madness and Social Bond, the Madness of Wars and Trauma*, in Athens. The speakers, Françoise Davoine and Jean-Max Gaudillière, were unknown to me at the time. Later, I found out that

DOI: 10.4324/9781003639022-1

Françoise Davoine and Jean-Max Gaudilliere were professors at the Ecole Des Hautes Etudes en Sciences Sociales in Paris, and they investigated the ruptures in what they have termed "the social link."

Their thought is of particular interest for this book on "Psychoanalysis and Refugees" as they conclude – as I concluded from my work with refugees and their carers – that "the classical opposition between cognitive knowledge and unconscious knowledge is put in question" ... and that "cognitive issues connected with sociohistorical realities and the attendant emotions are accessible only via the transference" (Reis 2007, 623).

So, let us go back to 1998. Beginning their speech, they asked the audience: "Are you sufficiently aware of the history of Greece, its connections with your personal history, and the meeting points with the history of your patients' homeland and the connections with their personal history?"

The beginning of the speech with a personal question was very different from what I expected. Something in the tone and directness of the utterance conveyed that it was not a rhetorical question, but the speaker actually expected us to answer it. I perceived in me a dysphoric and slightly angry reaction: "But we do not have wars in Greece. We live in a peaceful corner of the planet." Nonetheless, the speaker continued: "And if you do not have wars now, do you know how your parents and/or your grandparents experienced the war? Have you ever considered the impact of your country's history on your ancestors and yourselves?"

Soon I realized that I avoided from the beginning to connect experientially with the topic of the speech; I wanted to escape "meeting" the war by pretending to be "mad" like Odysseus in the tragedy mentioned in Kohut's last lecture (1981):

> Palamedes, Menelaus, and Agamemnon went to summon Odysseus to the Trojan War. However, the king of Ithaca, not wanting to follow them, pretended to be mad. Having yoked an ox and a horse in the plow, he sows salt instead of seeds. Then, the imaginative Palamedes put baby Telemachus in front of the plow. Odysseus makes a semicircle to avoid him, thus revealing his mental health and consequently accepting to go to war.

Kohut calls the above semicircle the *"semicircle of mental health,"* emphasizing that it determined the future of the father–son relationship (Kohut 1981): Telemachus not only searches for his father but is by his side an ally and companion in the final battle against Penelope's suitors. Winning this battle, Odysseus regains his wife and his throne in Ithaca. Odysseus and Telemachus are a father–son pair different from the well-known psychoanalytic pair of Father Laius and his son Oedipus.

It has been a long time since 1998; in the meantime, I have dealt with madness, trauma, and refugees in different contexts. However, the listeners' reaction to a similar question to the one posed by the two psychoanalysts in 1998 is the same; it seems to entail an avoidance of the thought of war.

Silence and Acknowledgment

It often seems that the psychoanalytic mind is expected to preoccupy itself with issues regarding family relations, such as how much a father hates his child, like Laius hates Oedipus. What might a psychoanalyst find interesting in the fields of war and refugees?

Ghislaine Boulanger referred to a similar silence when she asked the advanced candidates at an analytic institute if they could offer examples from their own practices to illustrate cases of adults who had been traumatized as adults. "When I asked about examples of catastrophic stress in adulthood, there was silence. No one even asked me what I meant" (Boulanger 2007, 2). Boulanger's lecture was able to remove the trainees' initial silence. As she started to present her theory on understanding and treating *Adult Onset Trauma*, the candidates who were first shocked recognized that they had such cases in their current practices – at least half of the seminar members (Boulanger 2007, 2).

Among the ways to learn (theoretically, practically, and experientially), the most important in the psychoanalytic perspective, the one that organizes the others, is *experience*. In his book *The Body Keeps the Score*, Bessel Van Der Kolk refers to his teacher, Elvin Semrad, who taught them to be wary of psychiatry textbooks. He wrote that therapists' job is to help people acknowledge, experience, and bear the reality of life with all its pleasure and heartbreak. "The greatest source of our suffering is the lies we tell ourselves" (Van Der Kolk 2014, 26).

Then, what can we do? Is it better to recommend to caregivers of refugees that they rely on their empirical knowledge or provide them with certain theoretical and clinical material? Can we help them gain personal experience by providing them with theory? We have the tools but not the theory, claims Boulanger in the above-mentioned book. In my book, I tried to do my own research on how we can dive into our emotional reactions to try to restore the "ruptures in the links."

I think this is what both Boulanger – on the above occasion – and Davoine – in her speech in 1998 – achieved when she put as another Palamedes in front of "my plough," my loved ones. What I experienced listening to Françoise Davoine's speech created bonds of communion with my ancestors and my patients. For example, when I heard about the ritual framework of the Plains Indians, where one is not accepted only as an individual but in the name of all that one is related to (all my relatives) (Davoine and Gaudillière 2004, 26), I thought of my ancestors affected by war and refugee. I remembered my grandfather crying while singing in Turkish – Turkish was and is a foreign language unknown to me – during holidays. From my grandfather, I passed by association to my father and uncles, who cried after their father's death, singing in the same Turkish language that I did not understand, but that overwhelmed me with sadness and nostalgia.

Boulanger cites the two French psychoanalysts who emphasize the further dangers of not recognizing and treating adult-onset trauma. She supposes that perhaps, being *French psychoanalysts*, "they had too many opportunities to analyze previously unrecognized wartime trauma as it precipitates out during the treatment of a daughter or a grandson" (Boulanger 2007, 5).

However, my understanding of their theory is that there is not a single corner of the planet where one cannot detect significant disasters in various generations, whether recent or remote. Can madness in a psychotic patient be connected to the wars of his ancestors? Perhaps there is no final answer to this question, but in order to search for the connection between madness and trauma, we have to turn our attention to the transference and the countertransference. In other words, we have to recognize our defense mechanisms (such as denial or disavowal) and our limits genuinely without abandoning the traumatized person.

For example, how can I think of the words of a psychotic patient of mine from Armenia who shouted angrily: "We do not speak the same language?" What emotional reaction gave rise to me? The fact is that he was fluent in Greek since he was a third-generation refugee. Did the fact that I, too, was a third-generation refugee in my country play a role in denying the connection between his madness and Armenian history, avoiding the pain of the persecution of the Armenians? Was it my defense not to want to know about the disaster that led me not to care about what he was telling me?

Françoise Davoine's talk rekindled my interest in meeting my psychotic patients and trying to "understand" their madness. I wondered for some years how to think about schizophrenic speech and, above all, about the experience of meeting an individual with some kind of psychotic disorder. During this process, I noticed that when I talked about my schizophrenic patient in any group of colleagues, my interlocutors found the narrative interesting. Nonetheless, I was not able to put into words anything of my – almost – innate strong defensive impulse to leave the meeting with the schizophrenic person. Did such an experience during the encounter with a psychotic person require literary talent to be told that I did not possess? And then again, maybe the literary talent destroys schizophrenic speech at its essence? Would it organize it, direct it toward a goal, and madness would no longer be recognizable? I already knew how careful I ought to be with the claim of understanding psychotic speech.

However, Davoine and Gaudilliere were telling me *to understand myself.* Gerard Fromm, director of the Erikson Institute/Austen Riggs Center, prefacing the book *History and Trauma* (Davoine and Gaudilliere 2004), repeated the phrase: "If for whatever reason excluded stories cannot be transmitted in a verbal form given by the person who experienced them, they will be narrated by another." He wanted to underline the necessity of "putting into words" of telling the excluded stories (Fromm 2003).

Starting the Journey

With two or three colleagues, we started going to Paris to present a clinical case of a psychotic patient to Françoise Davoine and Jean-Max Gaudilliere. They invited us to participate in their seminar at the Ecole des Hautes Etudes en Sciences Sociales (EHESS). In July 2001, two of us took part, together with about 20 guests from Europe, North America, and South America, in a workshop entitled "Casus Belli."

The guests were invited to present, taking the floor spontaneously, a turning point in the axis of the transference and countertransference of psychotic patient treatment, linking it to a broader social and historical trauma. As Gerard Fromm wrote, it was important that we did not introduce ourselves through our official titles but based on a point in our relationship with our patient that led one to present his case spontaneously after another. It was as if we let our unconscious choose the connection to what preceded.

We tried to create moments of connection in stories of disconnection. This first meeting, which gave rise to the aforementioned book *History and Trauma*, was followed by a second one in Greece, on the island of Tinos, entitled "Casus Belli 2," based on the same logic as the previous one. In "Casus Belli 1," I presented the case of an 18-year-old young girl whose "madness" turned out, after several years of treatment at the pace of two sessions weekly, to be in remarkable symmetry with traumatic events of her early adolescence. Her delirium and hallucinations were associated with the traumas of her biography. The removal from her home and the internal migration for study purposes (a frequent cause of *interior migration*[1] in Greece, where universities are concentrated in the big cities) caused the further dismantling of the boundaries of her ego and the inability to metabolize and control her emotions, resulting in the psychopathological image of psychosis that led her to treatment. Auditory hallucinations, insomnia, agitation, impairment of her functionality in her studies but also in the ability to take care of her hygiene, and delirium of reference to herself with a persecutory tone led her to my office.

Years later, I discovered that her psychotic symptoms "spoke out" the trauma of an incestuous, two-year love affair in her early teens, which was revealed by an unwanted pregnancy. The denial, the refusal of the parents regarding the recognition of the abusive behavior of the adult relative and instead the punishment of Niki in various ways led her to a psychotic experience of herself and reality, which she could hide adequately for years.

Suppose one wonders about the connection with the social level. In that case, it is enough to consider that in the case of Niki, the denial of domestic violence was the result of trauma not only to her but also to her family through "shame" (I will present similar incidents of abuse of women and coping with shame in refugee women). The family felt stigmatized, defiled, and unacceptable within the village community. Shame, a powerful emotion, as we will also see in the cases of refugees I present in this book, led to Niki's lack of legal protection. Despite the undeniable pregnancy, the abuser and his wife reacted with threats against Niki when she named him responsible. This is the perverse distortion that is often observed in different religious and social traditions: the perpetrator is acquitted, and the victim must "disappear in one way or another" for shame to be washed away.

Returning to the Future

The denial of extreme violence is observed beyond individual cases, in collective cases of trauma, in political and social phenomena, in history. In the case of collective trauma, replacing the attitude of denial as early as possible with acknowledging what happened or is happening is a key step toward healing the victim – or victims. *Acknowledgment* is an attestation of receipt, an acceptance that something *did* happen, while denial is experienced as an additional trauma, an experience of betrayal. In the above case, the representation of a world dominated by law is torn to pieces. For example, it may equally be detected in the victims who were tortured by the police of the Pinochet regime in Chile, where society is silent in the face of the initial trauma. The torturer also may deny (or/and possibly enjoy) the pain he inflicts on the victim (Benjamin 2018).

The result is that reality becomes an unsafe space, and words are distorted and lose meaning. In *"Talks on Psychanalysis* (2018)" (28:1 pp. 115–21), Benjamin uses the concept of *the moral third* to illustrate the position in which we experience the world as operating under specific laws. If we accept what happened, then it is possible to make amends in cases of significant trauma by acknowledging the harm and suffering it entails. When recognition of the trauma by the therapist can take place within the therapeutic relationship, it paves the way for the victim to feel secure about the importance and need of social *recognition*.

Recognition is the literal translation of the Greek word *ana-gnorisis*, meaning a change from ignorance to knowledge. The prefix *ana* implies repetition and the verb *gnorizo* is the act to gain *gnosis*, meaning knowledge. It is not by chance that Aristotle centered his comments on *The Odyssey* around the theme of anagnorisis. Odysseus is recognized by his dog, his father, etc. Papadopoulos cites Gainsford (2003), who identifies 15 such scenes. In each scene, a person recognizes another person. Papadopoulos reveals the

> insight, the epiphany, the new understanding that we acquire of a person, a place, an object, a feeling, or a situation that we already knew but had perceived in a different way. It refers to a renewal of an

understanding, to the second take of an already familiar perception that leads to acquiring new meaning.

(Papadopoulos 2021)

In such cases, the analyst functions as the witnesses in ancient Greece's ritual purifications, who watched silently as the priest washed water and anointed the defiled with oil. In an inscription from the oracle of Apollo found in the city of Cyrene, in the Greek colony of Africa, three ways of purification are proposed. In the third option, a mediator, a priest, and witnesses from those in public office in the city are added. A similar purification process is found in another inscription in Lindos and elsewhere (Robertson 2010, 353–54) a ceremony that was the exclusive pathway to stopping metaphysical punishment when the exile of the perpetrator or perpetrators was not enough. Witnesses could be perceived as possessing certain knowledge and a maturity of self-observation.

Witnesses' presence guarantees the proper functioning of the law, interpreting symbols and preventing the emergence of "monsters" that reside in the human condition.

Human violence takes many forms.[2] When someone is forced to flee their home terrified, having seen people they love die horribly, having felt helpless in forms of extreme exploitation and violence along the way, with no one welcoming them anywhere, being unwanted, unable to meet or recognize any "good enough object" to help them to recuperate, with their mind confused by constant obstacles, the word "trauma" fails to convey the magnitude of helplessness, weakness, and passivity caused. Regression and confusion make it impossible to perceive the new conditions in the places where refugees arrive. The above creates the conditions for a new trauma.

It has been observed that the shorter the time between the disaster and the cry of pain and despair that the catastrophic condition causes to the subject, the greater the chance of healing in the future. Therefore, it is important to take therapeutic action as early as possible. The time of therapeutic intervention in the refugee camp in Moria, Lesvos, can be one of the shortest in Europe.

Notes

1 Although migration proper occurs when the movement happens from one country to another, the displacements occurring within the same country could also be called migration in the psychological sense. We can use the term interior migration for the above move. These moves may be definitive or temporary, to greater or lesser degrees, for reasons of work, study, and so forth (Grinberg and Grinberg 1989, 17).
2 An immigrant leaves their country of origin in search of a job or place to stay in another country, having received the necessary documents from the government or embassy and is bound by the laws of the new country. Migration is con-

sidered a natural phenomenon, unlike refugee where movement is only done under violence or pressure. A refugee leaves his country of origin because of necessity or fear (avoidance of persecution, destruction of a home by natural disaster or war, violation of human rights due to race, religion, nationality, participation in a persecuted social or political group, etc.). Their rights are determined by laws, which do not apply to refugees, who live in camps, where they are provided with bare essentials and health care until they can return home or settle in a different country, with minimal rights under the Refugee Law and the 1967 Protocol relating to the Status of Refugees (Hein 1993).

Bibliography

Abraham, Nicolas. 1975. "Notes on the Phantom: A Complement to Freud's Metapsychology." In *The Shell and the Kernel*, edited by Nicholas Rand, 171–76. Chicago: University of Chicago Press.

Akhtar, Salman. 1996. "'Someday…' and 'If Only…' Fantasies: Pathological Optimism and Inordinate Nostalgia as Related Forms of Idealization." *Journal of the American Psychoanalytic Association* 44 (3): 723–53.

Bazaridis, Konstantinos. 2023. "Talking about the Father." In *The Father: Psychoanalytic Perspectives*, edited by Luigi Zoja. Athens: Armos Publications.

Benedetti, Gaetano. 1998. *Le Sujet Emprunté: Le Vécu Psychotique du Patient et du Thérapeute*. Paris: Éditions Érès, Collection La Maison Jaune.

Benedetti, Gaetano. 2002. *La Psychothérapie des Psychoses Comme Défi Existentiel*. Paris: Éditions Érès, Collection La Maison Jaune.

Benjamin, Jessica. 2018. "How Therapy with Victims of Political Trauma Repairs the Third: Commentary on Gómez and Kovalskys's Work in the Context of Post-Dictatorship Chile." *Psychoanalytic Dialogues* 28: 115–21.

Boulanger, G. 2007. Wounded by Reality. Psychology Press. Taylor and Francis Group. New York, London. Copyright by The Analytic Press (2007). Published in 2009 by the Psychology Press.

Bromberg, Philip. 2003. "One Need Not Be a House to Be Haunted." *Psychoanalytic Dialogues* 13: 689–709.

Caruth, Cathy. 1996. *Unclaimed Experience*. Baltimore: Johns Hopkins University Press.

Cassin, Barbara. 2013. *La Nostalgie: Quand Donc Est-On Chez Soi? Ulysse, Énée, Arendt*. Paris: Éditions Autrement. Trans. into Greek by Cécile Inglessi-Margelou. 2015. Athens: Ink.

Christopoulou, Anna, Giannoulaki Chrysi, and Tzavaras, Nikos. 2023. "Mourning and Identity Issues in the Treatment of Refugees in Lesvos." In *Trauma, Flight, and Migration: Psychoanalytic Perspectives*, edited by IPA in the Community, London and New York: Routledge.

Davoine, Françoise. 2007. "Reply to Commentaries." *Psychoanalytic Dialogues* 17: 671–682.

Davoine, Françoise, and Jean-Max Gaudillière. 2004. *Histoire et Trauma*. Trans. into Greek by Kounezis, Marina, curated by Gkiastas, Yiannis. 2013. Athens: Methexis.

Dowd, Annie. 2010. "Review of *On Soul and Earth: The Psychic Value of Place*, by Elena Liotta." *Journal of Analytical Psychology* 55 (1): 139–41.

Eisold, Barry K. 2019. *Psychodynamic Perspectives on Asylum Seekers and the Asylum-Seeking Process: Encountering Well-Founded Fear*. London: Routledge.

Erikson, Erik H. 1956. "The Problem of Ego Identity." *Journal of the American Psychoanalytic Association* 4: 56–121.

Freud, Sigmund. 1917. "Mourning and Melancholia." *Standard Edition* 14: 237–58.

Freud, Sigmund. 1928. "A Religious Experience." *Standard Edition* 21: 167–72. London: Hogarth Press, 1961.

Fromm, Gerard. 2003. "Foreword." In *History Beyond Trauma*, edited by Francoise Davoine, Jean-Max Gaudilliere, and Susan Fairfield. New York: Other Press.

Garland, Caroline. 1998. "Issues in Treatment: A Case of Rape." In *Understanding Trauma: A Psychoanalytic Approach*, edited by Caroline Garland. London and New York: Karnac Books.

Gainsford, Peter. 2003. "Formal Analysis of Recognition Scenes in the *Odyssey*." *The Journal of Hellenic Studies* 123: 41–59.

Giannoulaki, Chryssa. 2023. "Is Psychoanalysis of Any Help for Refugees?" In *Trauma, Flight, and Migration: Psychoanalytic Perspectives*, edited by IPA in the Community. London and New York: Routledge.

Gilligan, James. 1997. *Violence: Reflections on a National Epidemic*. New York: Vintage Books.

Grinberg, León, and Rebeca Grinberg. 1989. *Psychoanalytic Perspectives on Migration and Exile*. New Haven and London: Yale University Press.

Grossmark, Robert. 2016. "Psychoanalytic Companioning." *Psychoanalytic Dialogues* 26 (6): 698–712.

Hein, Jeremy. 1993. "Refugees, Immigrants, and the State." *Annual Review of Sociology* 19 (1): 43–59.

Knafo, Danielle, and Marc Selzer. 2024. *From Breakdown to Breakthrough: Psychoanalytic Treatment of Psychosis*. New York: Routledge.

Kohut, Heinz. 1981. "Introspection, Empathy, and the Semicircle of Mental Health." In *The Search for the Self: Selected Writings of Heinz Kohut (1978–1981)*, vol. 4, edited by Paul Ornstein, 562. London: Karnac, 2011.

Layton, Lynne. 2006. "Racial Identities, Racial Enactments, and Normative Unconscious Processes." *Psychoanalytic Quarterly* 75: 237–69.

Leuzinger-Bohleber, Marianne, Gabriela Schlesinger-Kipe, and Nicole Hettich. 2023. "What Has Clinical Psychoanalysis to Offer to Traumatised Refugees? Some Experiences During the So-Called 'Refugee Crisis' in Hesse (Germany): Part I: The STEP-BY-STEP Project, Part II: Psychoanalytic Treatments of Refugees in Kassel." In *Trauma, Flight, and Migration: Psychoanalytic Perspectives*, edited by IPA in the Community. London and New York: Routledge.

Lichtenstein, Heinz. 1963. "The Dilemma of Human Identity—Notes on Self-Transformation, Self-Objectivation, and Metamorphosis." *Journal of the American Psychoanalytic Association* 11: 173–223.

Lifton, Robert J. 1973. "The Sense of Immortality: On Death and the Continuity of Life." *American Journal of Psychoanalysis* 33 (1): 3–15.

Lifton, Robert J. 1976. *The Life of the Self*. New York: Simon & Schuster.

Luci, Maria, and Miriam Kahn. 2021. "Analytic Therapy with Refugees: Between Silence and Embodied Narratives." *Psychoanalytic Inquiry* 41: 103–14.

Maronitis, Nikos D., and Loukas Polkas. 2007. *Archaic Epic Poetry: From the Iliad to the Odyssey*. Athens: Triantafyllidis Foundation.

Micco, Vincenzo. 2019. "Esprits Migrants, Esprits Adolescents: Transitions, Transformations, Migrations—Avancer sur les Marges." *Revue Belge de Psychanalyse* 15: 29–47.

Papadopoulos, Renos K. 2019. *Psychosocial Dimensions of the Refugee Condition—Synergic Approach*. Athens: Babel Day Centre, Syneirmos NGO of Social Solidarity, and Centre for Trauma, Asylum, and Refugees, University of Essex.

Papadopoulos, Renos K. 2021. *Involuntary Dislocation: Home, Trauma, Resilience, and Adversity-Activated Development*. London and New York: Routledge.

Reis Bruce. 2007. Witness to History: Introduction to Symposium on Transhistorical Catastrophe. *Psychoanalytic Dialogues* 17(5): 621–626.

Robertson Noel. 2010. Religion and Reconciliation in Greek cities. The sacred laws of Selinus and Cyrene. (AMERICAN CLASSIC STUDIES, 54). Oxford University Press. 414.

Van Der Kolk, Bessel. 2014. *The Body Keeps the Score: Brain, Mind, and Body in the Healing of Trauma.* New York: Viking.

Volkan, Vamik, and Elizabeth Zintl. 1993. *Life After Loss: The Lessons of Grief.* London: Routledge.

Film

Black Swan. 2010. Directed by Darren Aronofsky. Written by Mark Heyman and Andres Heim. Distributed by Fox Searchlight Pictures.

1 Language and Silence

The Question

I will begin with the key question that prompted this book: What can a psychoanalyst offer in a hot spot? Especially, if this is situated in one of the main entry points for refugees into the European Union during the refugee crisis, it means that, on the one hand, it may be better equipped, but, on the other hand, it entails an excessive number of arrivals. What can a psychoanalyst offer in space and time where refugees emerge half-drown from the sea, exhausted by a long and dangerous journey and where refugee caregivers – working either for state structures or NGOs – are also exhausted by the "impossible" task of caring for such a large number of people who are also injured physically and/or psychologically?

In other words, why did I, a psychiatrist and psychoanalyst from Athens, undertake to go to Lesvos every other weekend to support the team of caregivers of *Médecins du Monde*? Why did I want to be at the limits of Europe and at the limits of my field of knowledge and "my" native and professional language? How could I practice psychoanalysis, *talking cure*, in a Babylonia of nations and cultures where refugees, who come from different countries of Asia and Africa, speak many dialects, incomprehensible even to the interpreters who are the bridge between Greek and European caregivers and the newcomers?

As a psychoanalyst, I have learned to trust what relationships with other people will bring in the future. I have learned to endure not knowing the answers and to remain silent waiting for what my meeting with another individual will bring. I have learned that if I can provide a safe and supportive environment for the subject's self-analysis, for the investigation and discovery of himself, if I create an "embracing" environment, the desire of the other to understand himself and face the "monsters" that hinder his journey will naturally accomplish the rest of the work of healing (Winnicott 1965).

Nonetheless, what happens when the other is too exhausted to face the "monsters," when his psyche is "lethargic" or "dead" due to traumas too excessive for him? What happens when he has regressed so much that not only does he not have a coherent self that wishes to understand himself,

DOI: 10.4324/9781003639022-2

but he does not even have the symbolic "language," that is, *the ability to talk about* what he has been through? Or, when he does not recognize the boundaries between oneself and others, regressing into merging relations of self and object, because of massive regressive εmovements as well as multiple splittings and disconnections within the psychic apparatus? The possibility through the work of the psychoanalyst to bring about a change in the psyche of the analysand raises repeatedly the limits of language and its relationship with human nature and culture. Who will speak? For what trauma? Which body and when has it been injured? What language can "hold" such unimaginable pain and losses?

The answers to these questions are not as self-evident as it may seem at first. In the above cases, Freud and his *talking cure* meet Wittgenstein and the well-known quote with which Wittgenstein ends his book, the famous *Tractatus Logico-Philosophicus*: "What cannot be talked about, one must keep silent about."

If the refugee is seen as a multi-traumatized person whose "primary archaic trauma multiplied because at no point in his development or mental organization was he able to be fully metabolized" (Alexandridis 2018), what words should we create to name the people who arrived in Greece during the refugee crisis that met a zenith in 2016–2017, and what narrative to fit them into it relatively satisfactorily? I shall refer to a picture that Wittgenstein presented to his sister. The philosopher, whose insecurity had been adversely affected by the experiences of his participation in the war, had troubled his sister with his decision to become a teacher. It is from the greek translation in the trird chapter with the title Languages, in the second page there is a quotation from Hermine, his sister which begins; "his second decision to choose a totally trivial job and become a teacher in the countryside, I could not either understand it and etc" (Eilenberger 2018, 98). At first, I could not understand his decision to choose a trivial job and perhaps become a teacher in the countryside; and since we siblings very often communicate with each other via similes, I told him on the occasion of a long conversation: "whenever I imagined him with his philosophically taught logic as a teacher, it seemed to me as if one wanted to use a precision instrument to open boxes." To this, Ludwig replied with a simile that silenced me. He said: "You remind me of a man who looks through a closed window and cannot understand the strange movements of a passerby. He does not know what the storm is outside and how this man may struggle to stay on his feet" (Eilenberger 2018, 98).

Based on the above simile, the therapist must go out into the street and stand facing the one who fights alone, so that his movements find not an interlocutor, since the passer does not speak but a teammate or comrade-in-arms. Grossmark (2016) has written that the psychoanalyst becomes a psychoanalytic companion for people who cannot benefit from his usual interpretive activity. In this case, as I will attempt to show in the clinical material below, the change comes as a result less of what the analyst says or does, and more of what he does not say or do.

Psychoanalytic theory holds that for any encounter with a fellow human being to be therapeutic, the therapist must be ready to regress to the point of the fixation of the other, and therefore his pathology, is. The regression is perceived by the psychoanalyst who has learned to detect the movements of his psyche to understand the other, driven through understanding to exit the regression, hoping to gradually draw the other out of his pathology. The caregivers, wishing strongly, for different biographical reasons each, to understand the refugees, unconsciously regress and struggle with the wind and storm without consciously controlling this meeting outside the window, to refer to the Wittgenstein simile. In other words, the unconscious need to meet the other starts from different unconscious aspects of themselves or their ancestors and works by luring them out of the usual protective confines of Wittgenstein's sister's room.

When I was offered to support the team of caregivers of Médecins du Monde in Moria, I started out with a lot of hope: I had hoped to learn something more about my specific desire to go there later. Initially, I felt the need to encourage and support myself so I could offer the same to those working in Moria.

Of course, it was not just me who was mindful of a task out of the ordinary. Caregivers also, let alone refugees, doubted that psychoanalysis could help them. Nonetheless, at the same time, they wished that it could. It is characteristic what a psychologist who herself had done some psychodynamic work during her studies told me much later: "Our joke when a caregiver complained that he needed help because he felt exhausted was to say to him with laughingly, Like they will bring you a licensed psychoanalyst!" The wording reveals a deeper wish – that such help would be possible, despite ambivalence accompanied it from the start. This book aims at answering the question whether a psychoanalyst has anything to offer in the field of refugees' treatment and to strengthen the satisfaction of the wish to send psychoanalysts to this space – a wish that still seems difficult to realize for many reasons.

Clinical Material

Third Visit to Moria

I was already wondering during the flight to the island in what emotional landscape I would find myself within the group of caregivers. I had already read in the media about a tragic incident: a 6-year-old boy and his grandmother died from the fumes of a brazier they had in their tent, to keep warm. Then, a fire was caused by the brazier, which spread to part of the camp, without any other human losses. This was followed by riots in the camp and the decision to transfer the minors and unaccompanied refugees to another reception area.

Going to meet the first group of employees, I felt a pit in my stomach from the pervasive sense of sadness and worry. Therefore, I was surprised to be confronted with their *silence* about what had happened during the week and their desire, as they told me, to talk about "racism." In addition to the surprise, I noticed – feeling ashamed – at the same time a hint of relief emerging for the postponement of stirring up the unpleasant feelings naturally caused by the death of an elderly woman and a child just 6 years old who had been in Moria in search of a better present and future.

While observing the deafening silence about the violent death of the two people in the camp, I resorted to theory, as every time the situation is stressful. I began to wonder what defenses are used by the group – refutation, intellectualization, rationalization? I resorted to theory too soon, scolded myself, and decided to turn to "listening" to what the caregivers say, to catch the pulse of the group. Even in a crime novel the advice to the detective is not to look for what you want to find but to think about what you find – what it is about and why it is there.

A controversy had started around the value of offering education to refugees, starting with the fact that the two new tutors who had recently been added to the team of caregivers to teach Greek language to unaccompanied refugee children, were left without a work object, due to the latter's move out of the camp – causing them to fear of being fired. As their recruitment has been recent and they have not been integrated yet into the team of employees, they have been a convenient target of aggression that is surplus to people shaken by unexpected and violent events. "After all, we don't need them, we don't need what they offer," said the driver of the group's small van, reacting to the concern of the tutors in Moria. "Living needs come first, they are the urgent issue. Education does not matter if survival is secured," he continued with an anger that I felt was directed at me as well.

What do they need the supervision I offer coming from Athens for only two days at the weekend, when they and the refugees need a constant presence and help as they face death, medically imposed amputations, therapeutic pregnancy interruptions, endless mourning for untold losses?

I was not talking. I had already said to them the first time I met them that the goal is to speak as freely as possible, expressing feelings, fantasies, thoughts, events, dreams. The goal was not my answer or my knowledge, but the ability to better understand themselves in these traumatic conditions for everyone.

The discussion reached back at the Greek revolution of 1821 against the Turkish conquerors and the philologist Adamantios Korais (1748–1833), who advocated the view that the intellectual cultivation of the enslaved Greeks should precede the revolution, which he considered to have taken place untimely. The debate around the value of language (which was

Korais' main concern) and the value of politics in shaping the scale of values of what comes first and what follows to help someone in need turned into a fight. Like a fire that breaks out suddenly – I thought – and flares up uncontrollably.

A manual worker in the camp – who handed out clothing and blankets to newcomers – a local himself, from Lesvos, which is called the "red island" because of its significant percentage of left-wing residents – said sadly: "What do we have? We have nothing to give to these people! We have no culture, we have no laws, they are better than us!"

At this point, the interpreter interrupted him indignantly. A political refugee himself, he said:

> I can't listen to this anymore! I get incredibly angry! You do not know what conditions exist in the places we fled! It is nice to say all this but ask me what it is like growing up in a camp! There we were, people of many races and beliefs, benefiting from your country and your language. ... The greek we learned helped us great! I am here right now while other relatives of mine have died in the mountains of my country.

His eyes watered. "This is something that gives me no peace."

A social worker took the floor and said: "I do not accept this! I am doing my thesis on the differences of cultures and for me all people are the same! The concept of homeland is a stereotype, and I am against stereotypes!" The young psychologist sitting next to me whispered: "We are going to have a hard time here today." The interpreter continued angrily:

> Last time you said that refugee mothers do not take care of their children and now you tell me that all people are the same! However, at the time you had this derogatory style as if you were in front of savages: how can their child play with the wires and not be told "don't play with the wires, you could get electrocuted!"

At this point, I felt that I finally had something to offer from my psychoanalytic thinking:

> Apart from the differences that ethno-psychoanalysis studies in the many different cultures, there is also the psychic regression that takes place when one is in great need and this does not really change – it is something consistently human, an existential constant. Regression is a concept we use in psychoanalysis to understand what takes place in an analysis. The person in need seeking help is ready to regress to the most archaic stages of their psychosexual development – a regression that can explain some of the paradoxical behaviors of refugees in the camp. It is therefore possible that they feel too safe arriving here after

a long and dangerous journey. What can happen to their children in the arms of a great mother? They are safe now.

"Maybe!," continued the interpreter who seemed to want to attack even more the social worker "who is doing her thesis" and me for my theories: "But I believe that they do not pay attention to their children because this is what they do back home and in their village! They give birth to ten children knowing that five will die!" His position (racist and/or realistic) was followed by a muted, dismissive rumble.

The social worker took the floor again: "What are you talking about? What mother does not care about her children? Who gives birth to children so that half of them die?" "Mine!," replied the interpreter, adding

after all, they die themselves before they see most of their children die. I was a baby; I was only three and half years old when I saw her killed along with my father and older siblings. A neighbor smuggled me in Greece. It is a pity that I spoil your heavenly utopia for the human race.

There was heavy silence.

I thought once again whether I was wrong to take on this task that exceeded my powers. What could I offer? Those things about regression seemed truly little and intellectual. Useless information. I struggled to turn within myself to auxiliary objects, and people I internalized. In memories and clinical meetings. The ruthless, negative answer to my question of whether and how I can help once again darkened my psychic space.

While we were silent, I found myself reciting verses of the Nobel laureate, Greek poet Odysseas Elytis, from within:

They gave me Greek to be my language,
The poor house on Homer's sandy beaches.
My only concern is my language on Homer's sandy beaches.

(Elytis 1959)

Poetry as the last recourse? Is language, the last recourse, to the exiled, to the migrant, to the refugee a homeland that one never loses?

We came out of the heavy silence after some time with the psychologist sitting next to me observing in a spirit of reconciliation that there are nevertheless differences between peoples. You see that people from an African ethnic group are different from people from Pakistan. The reference to experiences with refugees warmed up the mood again. Everyone wanted to talk, they started from their observations about refugees and ended up talking about their own family and how in Greece mothers do not let their children move away from them. A young social worker said that luckily there were refugees, and he found work away from Athens! He was finally able to distance himself from his parents. He said he would never go back again. He is happy in Lesvos. A nurse from the island said that he would go to Athens to study and that he had now found the courage to come out as gay to his family and the local community. A nurse talked about the differences in the position of women that she observed and the importance of motherhood and about the thoughts that are caused to her regarding the demands that exist in Greece from women. One administrator said he loved that they finally got to know each other – half of them might not have met the other half at all until now, even though they worked for the same NGO.

In the end, one turned to the interpreter advising him not to take so much at heart whatever is said in the group since here he is not in danger of being "killed" because of some difference of beliefs.

The circle seemed to close with this conciliatory attitude, but nobody had touched upon the deaths in the camp. I felt that it is not good at the moment to do anything more than say how important it is that they have been able to speak freely feeling that they belong to a group, trying to understand what they are experiencing within it.

After the group session finished, one by one they approached me and told me that they really like where I joined them. They needed to speak freely and had asked for help, but they thought I would give them something like a lesson, like a seminar, and they had prepared six cases for me. Then the person in charge asked me to help them and see the six refugees psychiatrically. I was not hired as a psychiatrist, not even as a psychoanalyst for the refugees. How would those who had hired me in Athens react to this initiative? I felt that I could do nothing but accept. I also had to get out of the security zone more and even though my psychoanalytic Superego was "fighting" inside me that I would perform acting out. What would my fellow psychoanalysts say about such a faux pas?

Elements of Theory

The crude event in the above clinical material was undoubtedly the death of two people in the camp followed by riots among the refugees. The reaction of camp officials was to remove the most vulnerable groups of unaccompanied minors to better protect them. In the group of caregivers, no one talked about the fact of violent death and fire. They fell silent and I chose to remain silent too.

Why did I choose this encounter – and silence – as the first chapter of the book on refugees?

On the refugee issue, we are at the limits of language, transported to a disaster field.

The mathematician Thom (1977), who introduced the concept of catastrophe, defines it as the place where a function abruptly changes form, but he considers that there is no mathematical model that can describe the catastrophe itself. However, situations immediately before or after, are mathematically describable.

(Alexandridis 2020, 43)

I attempt to show how the psychoanalytic attitude contributes to the identification and modification of factors that without the latter lead to the repetition of a catastrophe, which on an intersubjective level (but also on an intrasubjective level) is expressed as the destruction of languages, according to Bion (the infliction of confusion of tongues) (Bion 1970). Not understanding languages leads to the destruction of Babel, an example given by Bion, among others, of the consequences of not finding a point of convergence to make interrelation possible.

Silence not only belongs to the analyst's arsenal but is imposed in conditions where tact and respect for human suffering lead to the realization of the tragedy of human existence. The act of silence (silence is an act in the sense of a conscious and/or unconscious choice of attitude of receptivity, passivity, and waiting for meaning to come at the appropriate time) is the space from which the connection of two or more people and the finding of meaning in the human condition will begin. With Wittgenstein's sister (Eilenberger 2018, p. 98), we have to abandon certainty to change our own perspective in a way to crack the window glass that separates our subjective experience from the experience of the other. Then the conditions are created for language to be able to act therapeutically.

In formulating the question, I referred to the position of Grossmark (2016), who claims that in cases where there is no differentiation between self and other,

the analyst accompanies the patient in dark, archaic areas of his functioning and regressive relations with the object where he is not available for conversation and interaction or for mutual inquiry, but seeks to provoke greater relationship and reciprocity in the encounter.

(Knafo and Selzer 2024, 62)

Frieda Fromm-Reichman has pioneered the proposal for meeting the regressed patient. In the book *From Breakdown to Breakthrough* (2024), Danielle Knafo and Michael Selzer cite from the clinical practice of Frieda Fromm-Reichman a highly informative example of how the therapeutic encounter between the analyst and the patient takes place – as long as they take place in the presence of the analyst. I will pass it on because it encapsulates the essence of my choice not to talk about the raw event but to allow the group to unfold without any significant interpretative intervention.

Frieda Fromm-Reichman had a patient in therapy who refused to leave his room or even acknowledge her. Not only did the analyst not abandon him because of this absence of his participation, but she brought a chair and sat quietly outside his room. This was done every day until the patient looked at her and asked her what she was doing over there. He was ready to start the dialogue (Hornstein 2000; Knafo and Selzer 2024).

What is illustrated in the example above is the need to adopt an attitude of waiting and preparation. Another image that helps illustrate the appropriate attitude is the image of Echo, who was content to repeat the words of the other without being able to say her own. Narcissus tolerated only Echo because she did not frighten him with her different "language" like the others who chased him, fascinated by him.

The counterargument, however, would be the following question: Did I have the luxury of waiting for the right time? In Moria, conditions prevailed where the next meeting might not take place. For example, an employee could be fired, another could resign, Moria could be closed, and another hot spot could be created, the government or the European Union could give the asylum paper to all refugees so they would leave the island immediately, and so on.

I talked about the regression taking place in the camp, offering metaphorical images and, hopefully, facilitating a first thought. In his second work, *Philosophical Investigations*, after 1929, Wittgenstein argued that language, through its inherent logic, carries within itself at any time, whatever the state of civilization, the forces needed to precisely heal those misconceptions and misinterpretations which it itself provokes and generates (Eilenberger 2018, 345).

I mentioned that the group closed with an "acting out" according to the psychoanalytic technique that would not allow psychoanalytic function to slide into psychiatric work. They asked me to function as a psychiatrist for refugees in addition to psychodynamic support for the group. In my opinion though, the catastrophic acting out had already been preceded by the operation of the camp – the expulsion of unaccompanied minors from the site. The officials aimed at protecting unaccompanied refugees without prior discussions and fermentation within the large group of caregivers (the many different NGOs and the employees of the Greek public sector) – a gigantic task, undoubtedly due to the enormous number of caregivers and the great differences between them. The right decision to remove minors was also a defensive tactic that prioritized an objective and measurable therapeutic act – thus diffusing a regime of constant anxiety in regard to responsibility management. This worked against an attitude of thinking about the discomfort, anger, and experience of destruction of everyone in the camp.

The splitting phenomena within the group of employees came as a consequence of a regression in ways of mechanistic and bureaucratic treatment of the destructive violence of fire and death. They were followed by the anarchic and angry reaction of refugees demanding security and justice – however, neither of the two was possible in the conditions of the camp.

How did these children and teenagers experience losing once again the place and the relationships they had created? The decisions made by others about us to be experienced as care and not as punishment, imposition, and subjugation presuppose a particularly good functioning of the psychic apparatus, with good differentiation of self from object. They also require an already established relationship of reciprocity between the participants, with respect for each other, a sense of security and trust.

None of the above conditions applied to unaccompanied refugees who, even if they had succeeded in the past to a greater or lesser extent in differentiating themselves from objects and abandoning to a certain degree archaic ways of relating to the other, such as merging or narcissistic perception of the other as twin, similar object (something nonetheless not stabilized due to their young age), they had temporarily regressed due to the difficult conditions of their situation as refugees. Would it not be desirable to avoid the violent movements and sudden and radical decisions that painfully penetrated their lives, upsetting the fragile balances they were trying to achieve? I shall write in another chapter about teenagers who are troublemakers, the so-called "difficult cases" that no sheltering structure wants them and do not know what to do with them. Their expulsion from protected structures places them as moving bombs in the social fabric that no one knows when they will "explode."

Returning to my third visit to Moria, the caregivers faced with their participation in an "impossible to prevent disaster care providing environment," regressed into a paranoid and quarrelsome splitting behavior. Because of their own threatened loss of their jobs, the two educators were closer than all other caregivers to the refugees' sense of destruction. In the group, instead of standing by the colleagues most affected, there was a very dismissive attitude toward the experience of the disaster that they themselves were trying to verbalize.

The absence of discussion in response to something so violent by care facilities has been observed to feed back previous mental injuries, resulting in the overflow of stimulation and violence in the face of an experience of suffering and a sense of helplessness. If the subject faces a support deficit that exceeds his ego's power to deal with it appropriately with his defense mechanisms, he withdraws from belonging to any group, and the pathological emptiness he experiences cannot be psychologically processed. Despite the splitting phenomena, the feeling of anger, and the misunderstanding that prevailed, freedom of expression was achieved in the group that eventually created a sense of "belonging."

In the support group, despite the silence about the violent event (and because of it), principal issues were highlighted, such as the following: psychoanalytic supervision in refugee structures, respecting the complexity of the operation of these sites, can contribute satisfactorily toward the recognition and processing of exceedingly difficult experiences, protecting the members of the group from mental fragmentation and burn out.

In the group there are representatives from various scientific strands and of different age, religion, and ethnic background. Each of the team members understands in their own way what is taking place in the camp. Devereux argues that there is a complementary relationship between psychological interpretation (involving an internal observer) and sociological explanation (involving an external observer) (Devereux 2015). The concept of understanding as opposed to the concept of explanation will be discussed in another chapter.

On the one hand, the communist wise man from Lesvos, who stressed that we have no laws to offer, highlighted an important aspect of the problem. On the other hand, young people came enthusiastically to work and offer to their fellow human beings, to teach them Greek and English, to help integrate into the new society those who obtain the coveted residence permit from the asylum service. The employees who belonged to the social fabric of the island had to face the additional fact that they belonged neither to foreigners nor to the locals, to the extent that as they were paid by the Greek state or by an NGO, they had access to benefits that the rest of the islanders did not have. As the elderly ladies in the village tell them: "NGO: month in month out, you have your one thousand euros. Why would you care about us?"

When I asked them how they dealt with this attitude, the field coordinator replied:

> I was invited to lunch yesterday and there were also my wife's relatives who are from Lesvos, and they were shouting angrily that they wanted the migrants to leave. I agreed. I just wanted to eat a schnitzel, I didn't want to sit down and talk about the refugee issue again.

The social worker sought in her argument the similarity and unity of people (a fundamental feature of mysticism and some religions, among other worldviews). The argument may have appeared naïve in that she supported it pseudo-rationally – based on the preparation of her thesis she demanded that her position be accepted, which was opposed by the group: "We all look alike, we are no different." But her thinking involves a critical issue that, despite the horrors of wars, remains always relevant to humanity. The universal need to resort to something irrational, deeply emotional that can be a peaceful refuge for a deeply traumatized subject. In the topic "archipelago," as expressed by DeM'Uzan (2005), along with the attack on bonds there is also the search for new self-calming sensations. The poetic element (like the ritual, the prophetic) is such a refuge. Language as a thing, as a sound before the symbolic function, is identified with the inspired and divine, as Plato put it: "The mystical element in relation to emotion, as opposed to the rational, is a universal aspect of human experience" (Hartokollis 2003, 226). Besides, being at the limit of the need to preserve my thought, I resorted to the emotion and evidence offered by literature and even more so by poetry.

Bibliography

Alexandridis, A. 2020. "War as the Basic Model of 'Catastrophe.' Ways to Think About 'Catastrophe.'" *Oedipus* 21: 35–45.

Alexandridis, A. 2018. "Palimpsests of Meaninglessness." *Oedipus* 19: 95–104.

Bion, W. R. 1970. *Attention and Interpretation*. London: Karnak Books.

DeM'Uzan, Michel. 2005. *Aux Confins de l'Identité*. Paris: Gallimard.

Devereux, Georges. 2015. *Ethnopsychoanalysis: Psychoanalysis and Anthropology as Complementary Frames of Reference*. Translated by F. Terzakis. Trikala: Beyond Publications. Originally published in the USA: University of California.

Eilenberger, Wolfram. 2018. *The Age of the Magi: The Great Decade of Philosophy 1919– 1929*. Translated into Greek by Koilis Giannis. Athens: Pataki.

Elytis, Odysseas. 2011. *Axion Esti*. 21st ed. Athens: Ikaros. Originally published 1959.

Grossmark, Robert. 2016. "Psychoanalytic Companioning." *Psychoanalytic Dialogues* 26 (6): 698–712.

Hartokollis, P. 2003. *Time and Timelessness*. Athens: Kastaniotis.

Hornstein, Gail A. 2000. *To Redeem One Person Is to Redeem the World: The Life of Frieda Fromm-Reichmann*. New York: Other Press.

Knafo, Danielle, and Michael Seltzer. 2024. *From Breakdown to Breakthrough: Psychoanalytic Treatment of Psychosis*. London and New York: Routledge.

Thom, René. 1972. *Stabilité Structurelle et Morphogenèse*. Paris: Inter Editions.

Winnicott, D. W. 1965. *The Maturational Processes and the Facilitating Environment: Studies in the Theory of Emotional Development*. New York: International Universities Press.

Wittgenstein, Ludwig. 1960. *Tractatus Logico-Philosophicus*. Translated by P. Klossowski. Paris: Gallimard. Originally published 1918.

Wittgenstein, Ludwig. 1961. *Philosophical Investigations*. Translated by P. Klossowski. Paris: Gallimard. Originally published Oxford: Blackwell, 1958.

2 Dream and Daydreaming

The Question

Refugees in Moria are admittedly arriving after significant disasters. Even if disasters lack the immensity that allows a refugee to get the coveted "asylum" (such as the war in Syria that caused a significant part of the European migration crisis), it is logical to assume that nobody risks his life on a dangerous refugee route (such as the illegal sea crossing from Turkey to the shores of Lesvos) unless an unimaginable catastrophic situation is underway. As long as legal pathways and routes of migration for desperate people seeking safety are not enough for those seeking refuge, sheltering camps for those entering a country without the proper procedures will continue to exist. As long as the camps exist, the need to care for refugees will pose burning issues.

Of course, refugees' living needs and health issues must be prioritized. Experience shows, however, that at this stage physical and living needs presuppose that the psyche must function sufficiently well to be adequately addressed. Can one deal with physical pain and seek proper medical attention when one feels "dead"? When he feels frozen and unable to feel his body as his own? The relevant descriptions are countless and enlightening. To illustrate my point, suffice to mention the case of a nurse in Moria who perceived the gangrene on the legs of a refugee who had just arrived from the stench, while the refugee himself was unable to ask for help. He sat frozen in a corner, silent and motionless.

With his literary prowess, Salman Rushdie described the freeze (of much shorter duration, of course) that grounded him at the moment he was attacked with the knife on 12/8/2022. "Why didn't I resist? Why didn't I run? I stayed there like a piñata in the air, letting him crush me." He wonders. "Was I so weak? I was such a fatalist." And then again: "Why didn't I react? I do not know what to think and how to answer. Some days I feel embarrassed and even ashamed because I did not resist" (Rushdie 2024). Suppose someone who can self-observe and manage the word like Rushdie does not know how to respond! Consequently, we can imagine what happens to the mind of people who are in danger of dying for much longer than the 27 seconds that lasted the deadly attack on the famous writer – we

DOI: 10.4324/9781003639022-3

leave out here the added trauma of fatwa (religious decree ordering his assassination) by Ayatollah Khomeini who persecuted him for 33 years and six months! Moreover, in Rushdie's case, many of the listeners present, starting with Henry Reese, the creator of the City of Pittsburgh Asylum program, reacted – in Rushdie's place? – by immobilizing the assailant until security men caught him. If we think of those present as a helping ego of the frozen Rushdie – a self-object performing a function in his place – we have a representation of how a parent acts on behalf of his baby when it still cannot act; how he saves the life of the infant while still unable to survive on its own. For years, the child survives because the parent is there for him.

According to the Freudian main theory of the psychic apparatus, the infantile element is maintained within the adult. Psychoanalytic theories resort to early childhood, the archaic, the primary for the understanding of human psychopathology, and the corresponding conception of therapeutic action. For example, for Mahler, the development of a healthy sense of self is intertwined with the provision by the mother to the child of appropriate experiences of symbiotic fusion and differentiation. Continuous and periodic returns to this merger are essential (Mahler, Pine, and Bergman 1975). Loewald (1960) emphasizes the parental organization of the child's experience, which the child gradually learns to do for himself, through identification with the parent. Winnicott (1971) and Kohut (1973) are the two psychoanalysts par excellence who conceived coherent theories centered on creating a living and true self as the prominent issue of early childhood. Bion (1957) refers to a similar view of man – the organization of the archaic experiences of the child by the mother and her functions that thus become the "content" of the child. In all the above theories, the organization of the child's experience is mediated by the experience of the mother.

Why are we interested in the above consideration at this point? How does it help us to face the question: "How can we act therapeutically in an EU refugee entry center?" A metaphorical way to conceive of how the therapist acts in cases of urgency, such as the Moria camp or Rushdie's assassination attempt, is to perceive the therapist's mind moving in a manner analogous to the mother in the archaic period of the child's life. Of course, the above view is not a scientific discovery but should be understood as a *proposal*. As for me, I was eager to assess a research method that highlights the particularity of each individual and collective history and links its understanding to psychoanalytic theories. It remains for the reader and future researchers to evaluate its effectiveness and reliability.

Based on the above view, creating a relationship with the characteristics of the mother–infant relationship is therapeutic, where the mother becomes the content of what the infant cannot experience by connecting the infant with representations that represent it. The above connection is a condition sine qua non for transforming experiences into psychic material about which one can talk later, when, and to whomever one wants. However, this relationship is one of great trust. The difficulty in the refugee field lies in the fact that trauma makes it difficult to establish not only close interpersonal relationships but also any kind of relationship, leading the refugee to the desire to isolate and disconnect. For example, how can one get out of their tent and watch the children in Moria play when one leaves one's home at night, leaving one's children defenseless against the vengeful fury of one's husband and their father? I will refer to this woman in the clinical material below. For this purpose, I will give her a name. I chose *Maryam*, which means *beloved*. The connection with the heroine in Toni Morrison''s novel *Beloved* is not a random one. Although of varying extent and intensity, the despair and murderous violence of the heroine of the Nobel Prize-winning author – the story is based on actual events – who killed her child to save it from the horrors of slavery, has common points with Maryam. In an inhumane and profoundly sick environment, the deviant behavior of a mother who kills or abandons her children can be seen potentially as a cry in the direction of life that seeks to be heard as a normal and healthy rebellion response.

The experience of psychoanalysts who have worked in refugee camps has shown – and my experience has confirmed this – that not only refugees but also caregivers are skeptical and reluctant to psychoanalytic help. The distrust is usually expressed tacitly and unconsciously with questions such as "Will you help me or take advantage of me?" "I need you. Will you always be there?" "If I turn my trust and hope to you, will you not disappoint me, or will the disappointment be tolerated?" Mistrust is more intense when the therapist is "foreign" to the individual or group.

Stepping outside the usual conditions of psychoanalytic work, however, I become a "foreigner" not only for caregivers and refugees in Moria but also for colleagues in Athens. I have spoken about Maryam in at least two clinical meetings: one in a psychoanalytic circle and the other in a broader milieu. In both cases I felt "alienated" and ashamed of the little scientific interest such a simple recording could have. After all, what did I have to present? Two encounters with a woman in Moria who told me her nightmares. Moreover, this woman, as one listener, a respected and experienced psychoanalyst himself, told me, "she was a borderline patient already before the refugee journey. Otherwise, she would not have left her children to save herself." Was he right? Probably. I detected within me feelings of shame about Maryam's attitude and guilt about my inability to defend her better publicly. Then I realized that I shared the same feelings with her – sentiments of shame and guilt as she felt powerless to defend her children.

Were my feelings of shame and inadequacy mine only, or did other caregivers feel them too? Were they part of the traumatic condition, so they pointed in the direction of the possibility of healing? Would it not be good to think about them and try to put them into words? Should I talk about my inner cry of despair because of the inability to function in the – helpful, as I have concluded – way I have learned to act in my usual working conditions?

It has been observed that the shorter the time between the disaster and the cry of pain and despair that the catastrophic condition causes to the subject, the greater the chance of healing in the future. It is crucial to take therapeutic action with refugees as early as possible. The time of therapeutic intervention in the refugee camp at their place of entry is the minimum within European territory. In addition, the extent of the disasters that have already marked them creates a situation of "urgency," which is the focus of the first part of this book.

Clinical Material

When Maryam, 22 years old, came to the MDM (Médecins Du Monde) clinic in Moria in December 2016 after her third suicide attempt, the psychologist who had treated her became alarmed and referred her to me for psychiatric evaluation. Maryam did not talk about a "suicide attempt"; she talked about the many pills she took to sleep and rest. Her problem was that she was constantly having nightmares and was afraid to sleep – nightmares and insomnia are among the most common symptoms of refugees in Moria.

The difference about the meeting with Maryam was that she made good eye contact with me and did not look at the interpreter or down, like most people the first time they entered the meeting place with the corrugated sheets for a roof. The eye contact prompted me to ask about the content of the nightmarish dreams that would not let her sleep. I asked her to tell me about last night's nightmare if she wanted. Maryam replied that the dream was ridiculous and meaningless. However, she could easily have told me because it was stuck in her memory, and she could not forget it no matter how hard she tried. She could not rid herself of the image of the dream. She repeated that she found the dream "ridiculous," before allowing herself to narrate it:

> Although the dream I had yesterday seems ridiculous, I will tell you. I saw a big animal and another small animal. The big animal looked like a dog and was wooden; although it was wooden, it gave birth to another small animal. Even though the little animal was seven years old, I felt he was twelve.

The brief time I had available in each meeting forced me to abandon my usual waiting position I kept in my practice in Athens with my analysands. I did not have time to invite her to free associations; I did not have time to indulge in the freely fluctuating attention of the analyst. What was left of the psychoanalytic technique? I seek within myself the bridge that was created spontaneously with the other, therefore unconsciously, as well as to add human civilization as the third interlocutor, thus, to "put in play" more intensely the preconscious part of my psyche.

My desire to communicate with her led me to the image that emerged when I heard about the wooden dog. Where else had I met a wooden animal? The Trojan Horse, as I had first seen it in a picture in a children's book, stood imposingly in front of me. Mythology is one of the primary areas where the psyche of the refugee and the psyche of the caregiver can meet, as many of the themes are found similar, albeit in different forms, in the myths and fairy tales of peoples. The admiration that accompanied my childhood gaze was helpful in the admiration that accompanied my look at Maryam, who could not help but intuitively grasp her. I did not find her dream ridiculous!

On the other hand, I recognized a shadow of resentment and a sense of betrayal stirring within me. The deception of the Trojans by the Trojan Horse. The deception of herself in the state of a refugee. The Beautiful Helen who so quickly left everything behind to follow the beautiful stranger, Paris. The grown-ups, my parents who abandoned me as a little child every night for places unknown to me. Parents and children. Treason. Deciding with a deep breath, I told her, "One wooden dog gives birth to another. You are talking to me about the birth of a child. You are talking about parents and children."

Maryam's face twitched in pain, and she said, "I have two children. My eldest son is seven, and the little one is three."

I thought the little animal in the dream was 7 years old: "You seem more concerned with the thought of your big son in the dream."

Maryam groaned and hid her eyes, rubbing them with her hands: "I really cannot rest! Nor should I forgive myself for leaving him behind! My son is disabled and was overly attached to me. I am afraid my husband might beat and abuse him to avenge me for leaving."

At this point, she cries and cries silently! I leave her even though the time is pressing to see the next patient.

After 5 or 6 minutes, Maryam says she could not even greet her children as she left. Everything happened so fast! She was taken away by her siblings, who showed up at night at home to take her with them on the journey to Europe! Her husband is a drug addict, and he and his whole family beat her badly! He would die if he stayed there.

She adds that she was told she could ask her children to come here through the UN, but they do not know when. She awaits for news daily and cannot deal with anything else! She tries not to think about it but gets desperate as long as she does not have a notification! Nightmares wake her up every night. She feels exhausted. He does not feel like he is human anymore. She does not feel alive! She does not know why she is doing what she is doing! She does not want to die. She just wants to sleep without nightmares, to calm down.

Me (thinking about the flight forward, when all this adventure and tragedy will hopefully be a thing of the past!):

> You wish your son was already 12 years old, as in the dream, to be stronger and cope with his father and the pain of separation, so that he can understand that you left but did not leave him and that you are waiting for him! And maybe then you will have already met.

I feel that she calms down listening to me speak. I wonder if I have the right to give her hope for reunification that I do not know if it will happen. I do not even know if her son has survived this father. However, simultaneously, her calming gaze makes me think hope is therapeutic! Besides, the corresponding UN Agency gave her hope.

So, I continued: "Maybe the UN will be the big wooden animal that will give birth to him in your new life, will bring him to you!"

"Wooden was the boat that took us from Turkey here," countered Maryam. She has the ability not only to agree but also to counter-propose. I thought she wished the boat would bring her son, but she unconsciously expressed her desire for the boat to delay bringing him by five years. She wanted to be freed from premature and unwanted motherhood. She was only 22 years old! I could not talk to her about her ambivalence at the first meeting. However, I chose to refer to the general cultural system that did not protect her but pushed her to such an early marriage.

> You feel guilty that you are no longer the one protecting your son. It is not your fault. You left to save yourself calling on your son to do the same and set an example for the little brother to follow when possible.

Time had long passed. Maryam left and asked me to write my name on a piece of paper to ask to meet me next Sunday. I am glad that we managed to meet at least for 15 minutes!

Theoretical Elements

I can speak from many angles about the meeting with Maryam. I will suffice to repeat at this point once again that the refugees, apart from being deeply injured, are also people who have managed to survive in harsh conditions, whereas many others have not. They are the survivors of violent disasters. The guilt of the survivor and the constant trauma of being treated as unwanted do not allow them to realize emotions such as pride for making it, joy to be alive, and/or hope for the future. It is our job to offer them. Acknowledging these feelings and what they have achieved and are accomplishing is part of recognizing their humanity and their need to maintain their dignity amid so many difficult circumstances.

Thousands of women are victims of domestic violence in Afghanistan. The media has many stories of women who were raped, tortured, and died at the hand of their husbands, brother, father, or by people assigned by the father or religious leader of the village to kill them to wash away the shame! Even if the shame had come from the rape of a 12-year-old teenager by a relative as she went to the field in the morning near her home for her physical needs!

However, I will add some thoughts that came to me when I saw the initial large turnout of people from all over Greece and Europe to help refugees during the explosion of the refugee crisis in 2015 and 2016 on the Aegean islands. I met people who quit their jobs and put themselves and their money at the service of refugees. This move is incomprehensible if we consider only the tragic side of the refugee's fate. The understanding that there is something bigger than personal history, an unfolding of forces around and within everyone, in which the refugee participates, fills every-one who participates – beyond fear or mercy and compassion – with that quiet pride and serenity that makes you feel deeply alive and human!

I will not dwell on these stories, which I consider particularly important that they are published! I will now return to the chapter's question: are meetings with refugees in an entry center such as Moria therapeutic and therapeutical?

Designating the tragic nature of the patient's experiences, Maryam's on this occasion, and the therapist's positive attitude to disaster create a bridge of communication that can restore continuity where disaster has created discontinuity.

The above position starts from the theory of Benedetti, the Swiss psy-choanalyst who dealt with psychosis and the psychotic patient. According to his thinking, each patient is a unique case where the human existential drama manifests itself unprecedentedly. I believe that not only psychosis, but any catastrophe can lead to another degree of the subject to an inability to think about his experience and his feelings, in other words, to a multifac eted splitting of emotions and thought. This splitting results in the negativ-ization of the subject's sense of self, which, to defend itself against collapse, is pushed to the archaic defense of withdrawal, which, on the other hand, further isolates the sufferer from the possibility of therapeutic intervention. Benedetti's psychotherapeutic method consists in positivizing precisely the negative experience that psychosis causes in the subject in diverse ways that we can see below (Benedetti 2002).

The positivity of a destructive experience is a possibility endowed to man's adaptive forces and, in a healthy person, takes place spontaneously. Van Der Kolk cites the example of the plan of 5-year-old Noam Scholl, who saw on September 11, 2001, the crash of the first passenger plane into the World Trade Center from the windows of grade A of the PS234 elementary school, less than 500 meters away. In the picture he painted on September 12 at 9 am, little Noam has recreated the image that has tormented many people who have watched it on television around the world ever since: people jumping desperately to escape the fiery inferno by gaining seconds before losing her life to the fall. In his painting, little Noam added a tram-poline to the base of the crumbling building. This is the positivization of negative experience, quite simply expressed. As Van Der Kolk comments, little Noam was lucky to have a safe haven in his home, where after he ran away from the disaster site, he was able the next day to make sense of what happened and imagine a lifesaving alternative to what had unfolded (Van Der Kolk 2014, 51–53).

The above movement of positivity cannot occur if the subject feels unsafe if the alarm bell does not stop ringing in his body and mind. An unexpected encounter with a person in the camp, a slight randomness, which makes possible a connection between the terrified person and a healthier psyche at that moment, can create the conditions for a positivization of the negative, catastrophic experience.

I chose the example of the 5-year-old boy I mentioned above because it consists of the positivity of an image. In the meeting with Maryam, I positively created the image she had created in her dream, but she could not think about it herself. Maryam's dream is a nightmare where her mental pain has undergone a significant degree of unconscious mental processing. Precisely because Maryam is capable of mental processing, she can, with my help, offer on her own the positivity of the association for the wooden boat that brought her to the safety of Moria. However, her psyche is overwhelmed by the discomfort caused by the experience she dreams of, the experience of abandoning her deaf child who needs her so much!

Maryam attempts to relieve herself by taking several sedative pills. The psychologist perceives this move as a suicide attempt. Even if she has such a dimension, Maryam shows her desire to live and wake up from the nightmare of being separated from her son in our meeting. However, the perception of reality is still traumatic and nightmarish. Maryam is not yet in a safe haven like Noam.

However, our meeting led to her asking for my name, which restored, at least temporarily, her mental function to the ability to produce thoughts on her dream that were linked to emotions. Maryam was able to cry by connecting not only her feelings to the thoughts of the dream but also having a witness who was able to make associations about her dream himself. What if I did not ask her about the nightmare? What if her dream did not bring me any association or emotion?

The experience of repeated dreams after psycho-traumatic situations indicates an obsession and resilience in the conscious effort of the subject to get rid of them. Bion (1962) claims that the failure of alpha function (alpha elements are thoughts that can be thought) results in the patient not being able to dream and consequently unable to sleep (Ogden 2005). For someone to be free of his nightmares and be able to sleep, the raw bits of experience, which are the nuclei of the traumatic nightmare (beta elements), must, through what Bion calls alpha function, become alpha elements. Is there any contribution from a psychoanalyst in just one meeting with the refugee?

Returning to the positivization of experience, a first movement of positivity is made through interest in the patient's biography, Maryam. To understand her dream, I looked for the elements of her biography; for example, she was a mother and had come to Moria, abandoning her family. Maryam felt that she was in a human conversation with someone who had a human image of herself and not just someone who was looking for the right medicine for her insomnia and nightmares. Another form of positivity is the therapist's ability to endure feelings of inadequacy or deadlock. The negativity of the patient, the impasse of his mental state, and the sense of persecution or emptiness that develops due to his aggression can cause the therapist's lack of interest in the meeting.

It is a fact that Maryam helped me take an interest in her through eye contact. But it helped me to take an interest in her (countertransferentially) and the interest of her relatives in saving her from the abusive husband. I could identify with objects in her life that cared for her. Most women in Afghanistan are not so lucky.

What led me to write this book, even though I am primarily a clinical psychoanalyst who works long hours daily with her patients and supervisors?

I agree with Ogden that writing psychoanalytic texts is a way of transforming psychoanalytic experiences that constantly push us toward reflection, especially when it comes to traumatic experiences on a microscale. What was traumatic was the fact that I was unable to meet Maryam again after she was transferred to another camp in the days that followed, so I do not know if she could find her son. So, I am left with the trauma of losing the relationship and wishing for a metaphorical "reunion."

References

Rushdie Salman. 2024. Knife. Penguin Random House. New York (p. 26 in the greek translation. 2024. Ed. Psichogios. Translator: Georges Blanas).

Benedetti, G. 2002. La psychotherapie des psychoses comme defi existentiel. Paris; Editons eres. La maison jaune.

Bion, W. R. 1957. Differentiation of the psychotic from the nonpsychotic personalities. In *Second thoughts: selected papers on psychoanalysis*. New York: Jason Aronson, 1967.

Bion, W. 1962. Aux sources de l experience. Paris: PUF, 1979.

Kohut, H. 1973. The analysis of the self. In papares on psychoanalysis. New Haven: Yale University Press, 1980.

Loewald, H. 1960. Internalization, separartion, mourning, and the superego. In *Papers on psychoanalysis*. New Haven: Yale University Press, 1980.

Mahler, M., Pine, F., and Bergman, A. 1975. *The psychological birth of the human infant: Symbiosis and individuation*. New York: Basic Books.

Ogden, T. 2005. L art de la psychanalyse; rever des reves inreves et des pleurs interompus. L annee psychanalytique internationale. 2005: 77–97.

Van Der Kolk, B. 2014. *The body keeps the score. Brian, Mind and Body in the healing of trauma*. New York: Viking. Penguin Group.

Winnicott, D. W. 1971. *Playing and reality*. Middlesex, England: Penguin.

3   Male Friendship and Homosexuality

The Question

> The experience of an eminently male environment, together with fierce emotional tension and, in addition to the experience of combat, provoke the manifestation of homosexual and sadistic impulses that would generally be suppressed. In the case of vulnerable men, that is, those whose repressed desires are particularly intense, this leads to mental breakdown.
>
> (Barker 1994, vol II, 154)

In Moria, refugees sometimes deal with experiences that seem incomprehensible and alien to them. The difficulty one has in feeling comfortable with oneself in relation to the social environment determines the degree of mental illness/health problems. "Am I crazy?" "Am I a pervert?" "Am I dangerous?" Many refugees struggle with similar questions, even if they do not talk about them, because they are ashamed. They prefer to talk about physical pain and any mental symptoms that show them as victims rather than perpetrators.

How does one respond as a therapist to questions like the above when these are expressed directly, as in Shayan's case? The differential diagnosis of whether it is a mental disorder in the psychiatric sense, or a peculiar, impulsive behavior arises as an essential question primarily for caregivers but also for the refugees themselves. The therapist's suggestion of a different, empathetic attitude is just as important as the differential diagnosis. The understanding and calm acceptance of the refugee's "strange" behaviors and thoughts can act as a catalyst in the mental processes of the specific refugee and all of the refugees and caregivers concerned by the specific case.

In his usual clinical practice, the analyst feels, experiences, thinks, and, at the same time, resorts to the theory that he carries within himself consciously, preconsciously, or unconsciously.

> Theory, which is the means for the psychoanalyst to understand what is happening, is initially a way of thinking that, in the context of the

DOI: 10.4324/9781003639022-4

therapeutic relationship, belongs to him and, during the analysis, is gradually allocated to the analysand too. In any psychoanalysis of a neurotic, the theory is a kind of "analytical third" (Ogden, Green).

(Vartzopoulos 2016, 215)

The issue in the case of refugees, and particularly in an EU first-entry camp, is that there is no time for gradual interpretative sharing. Can theory elements be verbally transmitted from the therapist to the refugee in the first or few meetings available? Is the above direct attribution of meaning to an enigmatic symptom for the refugee a tactic of "wild" psychoanalysis that will bring more harm than good?

Furthermore, is there time for the therapist to dither when there is a fear of a lethal passage into the act, as is the case with Shayan? When does the patient show that he is going through acts that escalate into violence and the threat of murder is expressed? Is it not a sign that the psychic functioning of the refugee operates on a preverbal level, and the rules of language cannot constitute and contain it? In this case, is it not important that the therapist speaks soon – here and now? Also, the risk that the therapist's countertransference will lead to an underestimation of the risk posed by the refugee's impulsive behavior is noteworthy. In the above cases, Searles' dictum on the psychoanalysis of schizophrenic patients applies, stating that the therapist, who will not act restraining with drugs and hospitalization but psychoanalytically, inevitably exposes himself to dilemmas and anxieties that sometimes endanger his personal existence and professional career (Vartzopoulos 2016, 216).

It is undoubtedly safer, in cases of need for urgent intervention, in order to avoid catastrophic multiple acting out, to cede responsibility to the effect of medicines. Besides, they referred many of the refugees in Moria to me, mainly for my psychiatric capacity and, incidentally, for my psychoanalytical one. However, is it not a perverse practice to medically "bind" refugees by silencing once again their desire, however unconscious, to express something of the violence and terror they feel? Of course, the question can only be answered individually, but the individualized response can be an example of similar cases, as Pat Barker's trilogy did for me.

Literary narrative can offer clinical diagnostic models to which the analyst can resort in order to understand his particular patient, especially in difficult encounters, such as individual therapeutic sessions with refugees. The excerpt I quoted at the beginning of the chapter is from the second volume of Pat Barker's *Regeneration* trilogy, the third volume of which, titled *The Ghost Road*, won the Booker Prize in 1995. In the second volume, titled *The Eye in the Door* (1993), Barker starts with the historical event where, while British soldiers were killed or were mutilated physically and mentally in France, London newspapers dealt with an article published in January 1918 in the *Imperialist* newspaper titled: *The First 47.000*. The author was Harold Sherwood Spencer, an anti-Semitic and anti-gay American writer and Captain in World War I, who convinced MP and publisher of the newspaper, Noel Pemberton Billing, that the Germans blackmailed 47,000 Britons into spreading homosexual practices in order to weaken British power. In a subsequent essay entitled *The Clitoral Cult*, he exposed many of the names of viewers of a private performance of Oscar Wilde's *Salome*. This was followed by trials and much publicity for the "sodomists of London" that drew people's attention from what was happening at the front and the absolute horror of death.

Before referring to *Shayan*'s case, where I will attempt to highlight the need for an intuitive conception of the problem and quick sharing of the conclusion with the patient, I will cite an opposite example from the psychoanalytic literature, which shows that the therapist's quick announcement of the otherwise correct diagnosis created fear and traumatized the patient. The analyst always attempts to move, paving the way for his intuition, but simultaneously subjecting it to constant questioning. The opposite example helps in this direction.

In the supervision of the few therapeutic sessions held at a counseling work center with students, Kohut highlighted as traumatic the premature interpretation given to an 18-year-old student by a specialist before she arrived at the center. The young woman asked for help because she lost interest in the subject of her studies and was thinking of dropping out of university. She also said she had struggled to feel good since her early teens. In time, she could have thought that the beginning of the discomfort in her biography coincided with a family move that resulted, among other things, in her father's change of attitude toward her. The professor's opinion from whom she sought help was at first that she was significantly involved with her father, and then a mental health specialist she later turned to told her that her father harbored Oedipal desires for her; their reinforcement in her early teens led him to project guilt on her for the retrospective perception of their previous tender relationship as incestuous. His daughter became an irresponsible being for him when she was previously a reliable partner. The interpretation, although correct in theory, was traumatic. It created in her great unrest, nightmares, and severe insomnia. She never returned to this specialist but also hesitated a lot to turn to a psychologist again for help. The theoretical correctness of the interpretation did not ensure the appropriate time and manner of formulation, so it worked traumatically.

Therefore, Kohut emphasizes the need to be sparing in what we reveal from our thoughts to those who ask for our help. Every psychiatrist or psychoanalyst knows and can say something that will both narcissistically impress and hurt a patient. He knows how to talk about the patient in minutes or even seconds, something that the patient has not been able to think about himself in his entire life. The idealization of the analyst is to be expected, along with a demand for immediate and miraculous help. The therapist should weigh the regression that will follow: regression is desirable, why, and to what extent? In the case of the 18-year-old girl, it was considered positive that the second therapist, when the girl referred to the controversial interpretation given to her by the previous psychologist, was content to repeat her words: there may be another interpretation. She did not seem to be in a hurry or desire to find the other interpretation herself. The attitude of trust organized the girl's psyche at a first level and time, enabling her to find soon female friends who could act as additional auxiliary objects (Kohut 1987, 203–21). The above example, of an apparently opposite direction to the one I will present, I believe ideally complements the thinking that should concern us in such cases.

Clinical Material

The 25-year-old Shayan (the name I chose means *"commendable"*) from Pakistan was referred to me because he constantly kept the medical and nursing staff of the camp busy with his attitude, something that made their already very difficult or "impossible" work complicated, as they were trying to take care of the multiple physical problems of thousands of exhausted people. On Shayan's last visit to Médecins du Monde, he said in a panic that he felt a strong urge to kill someone – which alarmed them – as violence in the camp among refugees is a daily issue. In their referral to me, they implied that Shayan was seeking attention, frightening them with his killer impulse, which, of course, was said with a negative undertone due to their workload with people facing critical issues. However, at the same time, they wanted the psychiatrist's opinion to ascertain that their assessment was complete.

Until the last visit, the caregivers thought Shayan belonged to the lucky ones who had been given a room in the city of Mytilene, within walking distance of Moria. He lived with another young man with whom he became friends. Therefore, the caregivers were not particularly worried about Shayan, considering that he would be one of the relatively "settled" and, therefore, calm refugees in the camp.

Shayan, a thin young man, entered the meeting place, his eyes lowered. He looked at the interpreter fearfully and, after some silence where he seemed to weigh whether or not to talk about something, he said he was asking for help to control some impulses that he did not know why they were occurring to him. He spoke fearfully but, at the same time, almost angrily. Shayan said in a horrified tone that he is not gay and that in Pakistan, he had had successful sexual encounters with women and did not understand what was happening to him. The point is that he gets into tender lovemaking with his roommate and friend, which has extended to other men, refugees, and non-refugees he meets on his walks in Mytilene. He spoke to the doctors, but they told him that a sexual relationship between two men was not a disease and there was no need to refer to them. They added not to be afraid because, in Greece, homosexuality is socially acceptable.

What was evident from his surprised and terrified tone was that homosexuality is not just unacceptable; it is something utterly alien to him. It is as if something crazy that does not stem from him is happening to him. At the same time, the interpreter translated the above with a similar expression of surprise and fear in his eyes; despite that, I had a subtle feeling that his voice was slightly wry. Internally, I felt annoyed having to expose someone who entrusted me with his mental world in front of another, who, moreover, was not able to maintain the attitude of self-control and neutrality, a fundamental principle of psychoanalytic technique, through the extraverbal messages he sent. However, because of the overwhelming lack of interpreters available, I could not avoid his presence or ask for a female interpreter who might be more suitable in this situation. Shayan did not know a word of English or French and, of course, no Greek. The issue of the presence of the interpreter and the impact it has is also a big issue in the refugee field.

I thought as I listened to Shayan speak with difficulty, awkwardly rubbing his hands against each other, avoiding my gaze and the interpreter's, often silent and breathing heavily, that he seemed a highly tortured man but neither mad in the psychiatric sense nor dangerous to kill. However, metaphorically speaking, I believe that he used the term "crazy" to characterize something alien to him that goes against the traditional values of the society in which he was born and raised and that he categorically denies its source within his psyche. Condensing what he said and organizing his interrupted speech, Shayan presented the following claims: "People like me must be destroyed. I am dangerous and immoral. I want to go to Mytilene and kill someone, but I end up having sex with a man, and this drives me crazy."

In the context of the daydream, I mentioned previously, Pat Barker's trilogy emerged within me, particularly the theme of homosexuality in soldiers. I quoted at the beginning of the chapter an excerpt from the talk of Wiilliam Halse Rivers, anthropologist neurologist, ethnologist and psychiatrist when he worked in a psychiatric clinic during World War I, with a patient about wartime homosexuality. I repeat it at this point:

> The experience of an eminently male environment, together with an extremely intense emotional tension, and in addition to the experience of combat, all this causes the manifestation of homosexual and sadistic impulses that would normally be suppressed. In the case of vulnerable men, i.e., those whose repressed desires are particularly intense, this leads to mental breakdown.
>
> (Barker 1994, vol. 2, 154)

The above theoretical evidence helped me understand what is happening to Shayan. However, what could I tell him that would help him? While I wondered what to say to Shayan, I was still annoyed by the subtle derision, a continuous sensation from the otherwise very competent and appropriate interpreter on many occasions. His attitude put me on my guard, and rightly so, as it turned out later. For now, I felt that this was an additional abandonment of Shayan by someone who could be on his side, and, obviously, I feared that his stance would be gossiped about among his compatriots in Moria. When love between men causes issues of life and death based on a people's cultural and religious superego, disapproving or mocking the "wrong or evil" kind of love is a way to make sure you are not in danger. I thought the interpreter could not help but have this mixture of fear and ridicule. Nevertheless, time was pressing. I decided that I had no choice but to talk to Shayan (and indirectly to the interpreter) about the need for "friendship" between men in battle or after battle, which could also manifest itself in the form of transient or more permanent homosexual behavior, often accompanied by particularly sadistic and violent impulses. I added that not only the condition that led him to leave his country (which I did not have time to learn about as he was overwhelmed by anxiety about what was happening to him in Moria) but also the refugee route itself is a kind of war, and a companion, like his roommate, is "a comrade in battle," with whom strong bonds develop (like Patroclus for Achilles, I was thinking).

I suggested that he take the time and see how his homosexual impulses would evolve after stabilizing his position with work and a network of relationships in Greece or wherever he finds himself. I also said that the violence of what had taken place in his life that I do not know (deliberately leaving undetermined whether he was a perpetrator or a victim) led him to think about killing someone. I asked him if he felt he could resist this urge by separating it from the urge to have sex with a man to feel secure and stable. Perhaps, in Pakistan, there were such men in his life that he now longs for them in the foreign land. Shayan had a small twinkle of joy in his eyes. He said he has four other siblings, all boys, who took great care of him as he was the youngest. They are all married and live in his village.

Shayan listened to my advice to give time and, most importantly, could perceive the emergence of nostalgia for the love of his brothers. I think he felt less persecuted by his homosexual desires because his Superego accepted nostalgia for the caring his siblings showed to him (and indirectly his father or mother?), so his enhanced superego power could at least momentarily control his Ego over his homosexual and sadistic impulses. My concern that a meeting was not enough made me want to add the necessary advice for safe sexual activity and the need for tests, but I reassured myself knowing that Médecins du Monde was very careful in this area. Shayan left with a slight smile on his face, which I thought was enough for this meeting, and able to contain his terror as another embrace. As expected, the interpreter, prompted undoubtedly by questions from others, disseminated in the camp what we discussed in the session with Shayan. Interestingly, my above interpretative stance circulated in the camp and led one of the caregivers to accuse me on my next visit to Moria of a racist and homophobic attitude. It was a sort of benevolent accusation that amounted to asking my views on homosexuality from someone who was fighting his own battle with his homosexual desires, but which were different from Shayan's.

For Shayan, I did not have any other information while I was visiting Moria, so I assumed that, if anything, his whole agitation did not lead to any particularly violent or delinquent behavior.

Elements of Theory

The act of violence and acting out, in general, often has a primordial symbolism that the perpetrator cannot put into words. Shayan fears he will commit murder and, at the same time, is both ashamed and boisterous of his homosexual behavior. How could I understand his fear of the violence that threatened to push him to kill?

The question that concerned me after meeting Shayan was whether I underestimated his aggression. Did I overestimate the internal reality where I recognized the attempt to talk about his "mental murder" and his nostalgia for his father and brothers? Have I been too influenced by the psychoanalytic theory linking homosexuality and persecution by paranoid ideas? I have been mainly concerned in my thesis with the Freudian stance on the homosexual fantasy of Judge Schreber, who suddenly, one morning, had the idea "that it must be something very nice to be a woman and to be subject to intercourse." Freud (1911) interpreted the fantasy as well as the dreams of the period when the judge sees that his old neurasthenia has relapsed as follows:

> At the recollection of the illness, the doctor is recalled, and the feminine phase of the fantasy is aimed at the doctor from the outset. The dream of the relapse of the disease means longing: I want to see Flechsig again.
>
> (Freud 1911, 42)

The question that burdens Shayan and Schreber is: "What happens to my body that wishes to unite with a man sexually?" The difficulty of both of them accepting it as they experience it, in this case, is related to the regression to the stage of narcissism, where tender devotion to the doctor is re-sexualized, Freud claims. Freud perceived a process of transference, which led the doctor to substitute another much more important person for the patient: the brother and, before him, the father. The defense against the homosexual attraction exerted on the patient by the men of his environment leads to a variety of mental expressions depending on the biography, personality structure, and ego strength of the patient.

As psychoanalysts, we have central to our thinking the importance of sexuality. Freud (1905) placed sexuality at the center of psychoanalytic interest by highlighting child sexuality as inherently bisexual and multiformly perverse – in other words, the child is ready to be aroused by anyone and whatever and feel its arousal through a variety of erotic zones (Freud 1905). The revolutionary thesis that the human being is sexual from birth created a rupture in the way man saw himself and brought Freud face to face with Vienna's scientific community – he was seen as a libertine who encouraged the out-of-law and moral expression of perverse sexuality (Gay 1988).

Psychoanalytic theory holds that we can organize the pieces of experience coherently and understandably if we seek the child within the adult. In simpler terms, while someone as an adult seems to us to be moving incomprehensibly, if we look at him as a child, his behavior is understood. If we also consider the knowledge of sexuality corresponding to that age, some light may be shed on the otherwise dark areas of his experiences. On this basis, we use the child's image as *a metaphor*. The analysand is not a child, but to think of him in such terms makes us find meaning and shapes in his experience, which otherwise remains incomplete and unformed.

The refugee, like any suffering person who asks for our help, regresses to the position of a child. He feels weak, frightened, and helpless, and needs to experience us as someone big who can help him. In other words, the refugee desires, fears, and experiences things as if he were a child. Even if he does not tell us about childhood memories as analysands lying on the couch do, we can perceive childhood experiences that operate beneath the surface of maturity, giving form to his feelings and behavior.

Due to the significant regression of refugees observed in Moria immediately after the dangerous journey that brought them there, when their Ego has not yet regained its limits, cohesion, and more mature defensive functions, their intrapsychic reality is mainly at the preverbal rather than verbal level. Correspondingly, the mental function of the analyst attempting to process phenomena of developmental stages that do not fit into the order of language/speech makes strong use of the metaphorical potential of language. In this perspective, the refugee is perceived as someone who needs specific parental functions, such as holding, mirroring, the possibility of a biotic fusion, etc. He cannot mature or quickly adopt Western European civilization's values unless given the right environment and time for internal maturation processes.

Our attitude of accepting differences without denying or idealizing them, nor wishing to correct them by exchanging them with our values and perspectives, is based, among other things, on the theory of narcissism. The introduction of narcissism was an important point in Freud's thought (1914). However, Heinz Kohut (1966) mainly explored its forms and transformations, as well as the feeling of shame that follows a narcissistic blow and paves the way for narcissistic rage in an attempt at revenge and a desire for magical reparation (1972).

However, the refugee is neither psychotic nor a child. Although metaphorical language helps us understand, we must not limit ourselves to this way of perceiving the refugee because the language will cease to function as a metaphor and turn toward a psychic reality. Metaphorical language is peculiar to psychoanalysis because psychoanalysis does not deal only with facts but with their imaginary interpretation and finding hidden causes that can only be implied. Since symbols or metaphors reveal the unconscious, psychoanalysis approaches the unconscious and tries to talk about it metaphorically.

Art and literature appeal to our intuition and thus connect the unconscious with the conscious perception. As I described in the previous chapter, the emergence in our daydream of heroes and excerpts from literature or art facilitates the intuitive understanding of the refugee. Freud often referred to writers for their understanding of dark areas of the psyche. However, he also sought to organize this knowledge and make it available intuitively and with clarity and precision. Could it be that the literature to which I resorted in Shayan's case was the result of avoidance of his feelings and thoughts, even if he could not express them in words, which led me to the pinnacle of violence that a psychoanalyst can exercise, the inability to treat the patient as a human being escaping any theoretical prefabricated conception? Did I resort to a ready-made according to the corresponding work of Marcel Duchamp? Did I underestimate his trauma and his personal itinerary? Did the rumors about the search for men for sexual encounters in a small place like Mytilene, which were already provoking derisive reactions in the camp, push me to a superficial, defensive approach?

Trauma is that journey between the self, others, and the powerful, Claude Barrois claims in his book on *Traumatic Neuroses* (1998, 172). Many traumatic neuroses are aggravated by the ruptures of a purely social nature that follow the first traumatic ruptures.

> It is as if every victim reincarnates the rupture of the social web… Psychoanalysis has the merit to be the only discipline that really does something: find again the trace of the point of rupture, a "before" where dream and fantasy had their place. Because death, his death, that someone saw face-to-face cannot be represented.
> (Barrois 1994, 73–75 in Briole et al. 1994)

Psychoanalysis has the advantage of being the only branch of knowledge that really does something searching for the trace of the point of rupture, claims Barrois.

When Barker's work comes to mind, it is also part of a context of discussions about the importance of male friendship in the war we have made with colleagues who took part to many work sessions on psychosis, amid which and in particular during one such session titled "Casus belli," to which I have already referred (Fromm 2003).

Ready-made inaugurates a linguistic function where before there was only an integration of Shayan's horror into something even more general and ready than my recourse to literature, such as the integration of his homosexuality into the way we perceive homosexuality in Western culture, which is neither his culture nor his peacetime homosexuality.

The friendship between warriors is a remarkable phenomenon related to proximity in battle, for example, the well-known closeness of Achilles and Patroclus in the *Iliad*. "The ritual doppelgänger deals with the body and soul of the other during life and after death" (Davoine and Gaudilliere 2013, 264). One cannot understand the closeness, the male friendship in war, if one does not know the loyalty that war favors. This friendship is in the etymological origins of the Greek word *therapon*, which arises from therapy, therapeutic space, and therapeutic meeting (ibid.).

At this point, I find the words of Hannah Arendt (1958) useful. In the foreword to *The Human Condition*, Hannah Arendt writes:

It seems to me that lack of thought – irresponsible risking, hopeless confusion, complacent repetition of "truths" that have become trivial and hollow – is a major feature of our time. What I am proposing here is very simple; it is nothing more than thinking about what it is that we are doing.

(Arendt 1958; 2020, 39)

We know that the philosopher who is interested in totalitarian regimes and man's forces of resistance to them seeks the forces of resistance in "thinking." Her meditation on "what is thought" takes a whole essay to approach.

As psychoanalysts, we know that in the treatment of psychotic as well as traumatized people, we refer to psychoanalytic theories and works of art not necessarily to understand and interpret but to keep thinking: to save our thinking from a stop that would be equivalent to our mental death.

Every attempt to think about a case naturally raises questions and gives few answers. It is, however, a comforting thought that the immediate response always runs the risk of aligning with current views and abandoning psychoanalytic radicalism. Hope consists of expecting each time that thought functions as a springboard for connections with other psyches in times and conditions when connections will succeed in the disconnections within the social relations network and the refugee psyche.

Bibliography

Arendt, Hannah. 2020. *The Human Condition*. Translated into Greek by Georgiou Peter. Athens: Patakis Publishing Co. Originally published in 1958.

Barker, Pat. 1997. *The Eye in the Door*. USA: Penguin Books, 1994. Translated into Greek by Katerina Kafourou. Athens: Odysseus. Originally published in 1993.

Barrois, Clauder. 1998. Les Nevroses traumatique, Paris, Dunod.

Briole, Gérard, Lebigot François, Lafont Bernard, Favre Jean-Dominique, and Vallet Dominique. 1994. *Le traumatisme psychique: rencontrer et devenir. Congrès de Psychiatrie et de Neurologie de Langue Française*. Paris: Masson.

Davoine, Françoise, and Jean-Max Gaudillière. 2004. *History Beyond Trauma*. USA: Other Press. Translated into Greek by Marina Kounezi. Thessaloniki: Methexis Publications, 2013.

Freud, Sigmund. 1905. "Three Essays on the Theory of Sexuality." In *The Standard Edition of the Complete Psychological Works of Sigmund Freud*, edited and translated by James Strachey, vol. 7, 123–246. London: The Hogarth Press.

Freud, Sigmund. 1911. "Psychoanalytic Notes on an Autobiographical Account of a Case of Paranoia." In *The Standard Edition of the Complete Psychological Works of Sigmund Freud*, edited and translated by James Strachey, vol. 7, 1–82. London: The Hogarth Press.

Freud, Sigmund. 1914. "On Narcissism: An Introduction." In *The Standard Edition of the Complete Psychological Works of Sigmund Freud*, edited and translated by James Strachey, vol. 14, 67–102. London: The Hogarth Press.

Fromm, Gerald. 2003. "Foreword." In *History Beyond Trauma*, edited by Françoise Davoine and Jean-Max Gaudillière. USA: Other Press.

Gay, Peter. 1988. *Freud: A Life for Our Time*. New York: W. W. Norton & Co.

Kohut, Heinz. 1972. *Thoughts on Narcissism and Narcissistic Rage. The Psychoanalytic Study of the Child* 27: 360–400.

Kohut, Heinz. 1978. "Forms and Transformations of Narcissism." In *The Search for the Self*, vol. 1, 275–303. New York: International Universities Press. Originally published in 1966.

Kohut, Heinz. 1987. *The Kohut Seminars on Self Psychology and Psychotherapy with Adolescents and Young Adults*. Edited by Miriam Elson. New York and London: W. W. Norton & Co.

Vartzopoulos, Ioannis. 2016. *The Common Origin of Logic and Madness: Psychoanalysis and Schizophrenia*. Athens: Potamos Publications.

4 Violence and Women

The Question

There is not a single person I met in Moria that violence does not seal their existence in various ways. *Being a refugee is itself a form of violence.* One does not leave one's homeland, one's natural and human environment, for trivial reasons. Their life or that of their loved ones is threatened, they have been tortured, they have been in danger of hunger and thirst, they have been politically or sexually persecuted, they have been or are mentally ill without the possibility of proper care, and so on. Even in the considered less violent situation of migration for economic reasons, I shall remind Gandhi's dictum that the worst form of violence is poverty (Gilligan 1997, 191).

Violence against women is a particular category of violence and is found in its extreme expressions among refugees. To understand physical violence, we must understand male violence since the making of "Manhood" is related to stereotyped gender roles, as Gilligan argues in his book *Violence*: "Men are honored for activity (ultimately, violent activity); and they are dishonored for passivity (or pacifism which renders them vulnerable to the charge of being a non-man (a wimp, a punk, and a pussy)" (Gilligan 1997, 231).

In patriarchal society, to the extent that women are considered to be man's possessions, they cannot have a will of their own and have no right to flee an unfavorable situation. If the woman questions her possession by the man, she provokes murderous rage against her because she takes away something that he feels is his.

In women in particular, narcissistic, often murderous, rage is directed not only by herself against herself (suicide), but often against anyone who is unconsciously part of herself (infanticide or infanticide). Freud has called the renunciation of femininity by both sexes the "rock of castration" (Freud 1937). Violence against femininity unconsciously is stirred in any man who fears becoming a "woman," for example, when he feels weak or feels homosexual desires for a stronger man, to become violent in order to disprove his feminine side. The need to disprove a strong, unconscious desire to "be a woman" is imposed upon men in patriarchal society by a

DOI: 10.4324/9781003639022-5

set of conservative rigidities and prejudices. In many countries of origin of female refugees, a woman's value is virtually nil. The woman is subjected to various forms of humiliation – in extreme cases, such as in Somalia, third-degree genital mutilation.

The most common form of humiliation of women is rape by one or more men both in her country of origin and during the refugee journey, but even during her stay in refugee reception camps. Even in the places of entry of refugees into Europe and in the cities where they are directed, the rape of a woman is, unfortunately, not a rare phenomenon and the possibility of preventing it seems to be very small. For example, as Swiss Teaching Analyst Barbara Saegesser, who has worked 15 years in East African cities, observes, many refugee women, especially from Sudan and the Kivu region (DRC), have narrowly avoided death and have been raped many times, brutally. The resulting narcissistic wounds lead them to think unconsciously, preconsciously, or even consciously that they are always asked for sexual intercourse in exchange for being offered a better living condition. This can apply to any relationship, even the relationship with the therapist, leading to the risk of being romanticized intensely with often unpredictable consequences (Saegesser 2023, 172).

Therapists, and refugee caregivers in general, in trying to limit the phenomenon of increased and continuous violence against women fall on a rock, different from the "castration rock" of Freud (1937), but immovable as well: the fact that a woman's silence and, often, masochistic acceptance of the need to buy her security with men's sexual gratification are the result of a long tradition of submission and shame. The emotion strongly associated with violence is the shame that lies behind many outbursts of characteristic violence called in psychoanalytic literature as *narcissistic rage* (Giannoulaki 2020). The shame of the constant humiliation to which women are subjected as second-class citizens in many cultures overtly and in others, such as the West, less overtly fuels the phenomenon of violence (Morrison 1989).

Psychoanalytic thought tends to delve into the far reaches of the spectrum of pathology or behavior (such as Schreber's paranoia) to delve into everyone's psyche (Freud 1911). In this line of thought, I will attempt, through the understanding of violence against a refugee from Tunisia, to delve, with the help of psychoanalysis, ethnopsychoanalysis, and literature, into some aspects of violence against women.

Before presenting the clinical material, I would like to mention some issues in the field of violence against women as the starting point.

Issue One: The ineffectiveness of measures taken to combat violence.

In an effort to find a more appropriate solution to the problem of violence, the causes of the failure of its treatment so far are explored by many, such as, for example, the psychiatrist James Gilligan, in his book *Violence* (1997). Gilligan worked for over 20 years as the head of psychiatric care for inmates in maximum-security prisons in the United States. In the above book, Gilligan highlights the unsatisfactory effectiveness of the measures that are still proposed today as appropriate for domestic violence. After important conquests (which I quote in a footnote), the number of women murdered by husband doubled (Gilligan 1997, 130–131).[1]

Issue Two: It is well established that publicity, instead of diminishing, increases all forms of perverse, destructive behavior against women and other groups susceptible to violence, such as children, regardless of gender, or transgender people. Jacqueline Rose, author, professor of humanities at Birkbeck University of London, and theorist on feminism, psychoanalysis, and literature, in her book *On Violence and On Violence against Women* (2021) refers, for example, to the release of the photograph of Angelina Jolie reaching out her hand to William Hague in 2014, saluting their fight against rape. Jolie and Hague aimed at, and quite rightly so, the recognition of rape as a war crime (2021, p. 36). In the Democratic Republic of Congo, where they focused their efforts, violence against women increased the following year and does not seem to have decreased since.

Jacqueline Rose argues that the following contradiction is one cause of failure. The particular woman who greets the end of this violence is the same one who repeatedly excites the viewers' imaginary love life through her appearances or films. Without fully sharing her position regarding the cause of the escalation of violence, we find it interesting to focus attention on the escalation of violence as a consequence of media coverage.

Issue Three (relates to the second): There is a behavior of spreading (through hysterical identification) the murders and abusive behavior described in the media. For example, an increase in murders was recorded in South Africa following the murder of lawyer and model Reeva Steenkamp by her paralympian and partner, Oscar Pistorius, and the publicity that accompanied his trial. Every 4 minutes a woman — often a teenager or a child — is raped, and every 3 hours a woman is murdered by her partner (in a 2019 investigation), while before the Pistorius trial murders took place every 8 hours. This phenomenon reaches such proportions that it is called *"serial femicide"* by Margie Orford, a South African journalist and author (Rose 2021). A similar increase in femicides in Greece followed the murder of wife Caroline by Babis Anagnostopoulos, a case that shocked Greek society in 2022.

Issue Four: The defense mechanisms of denying violence are an important part of the phenomenon. Tolerance and insufficient recognition of violence is strongly observed in the female victim, especially in the case of violence by the sexual partner. The above phenomenon is yet another puzzling fact in the field of violence against women. Violence is denied not only by the victim but also by peers and society, even institutionally. The victim woman shares the position of many of her fellow citizens, the police, sometimes also the judiciary, that the behavior of the sexual partner – behavior of belittling, social degradation and isolation, linguistic abuse, insults and humiliation, removal of all rights of protective objection, even physical violence – is an isolated incident that arises as a result of excessive love and devotion.

As an additional consequence of the above view, the use of the phrase "crime of passion" implies that it is something private, which concerns the relationships of the couple, and which furthermore justifies violence as an erotic outburst, thus excluding the wider investigation of multiple causes on which the social, cultural, and domestic timelessness of violence against women depends, along with, first and foremost, the perpetuated male "superiority" (Laufer and Ayouch 2018). However, research shows that the cycle of violence is far from isolated incidents, therefore often the word passion and the word love can obscure and work against preventing women's emancipation and for oppressing women's sexuality (Cooke 2022).

The denial of violence by and against our most loved ones is dictated by our need to preserve our faith in idealized conceptions of ourselves and others. It has been a point of criticism that Freud himself refuted the violence of parents against their children when he abandoned the first theory of trauma (Masson 1985). The shift to focus the root of violence from the external environment on the child itself and its internal, impulsive life has been seen by later psychoanalysts as a defensive attempt to rescue not only the perverse father of trauma theory, but his idealized mother too (Atwood and Stolorow 1993, 43).

Issue Five: The Silence of the Victims (Gammeltoft 2016): Simply put, the main question is formulated as follows: Why do women enter into relationships that are violent in many different ways in the first place and choose to remain silent for years (Snider 2018)? The clinical material contributes significantly to the understanding of the silence of victims of violence as a manifestation of post-traumatic syndrome that lasts an indefinite period of time –possibly for the entire life of the victim, if no treatment intervenes (Garland 1998).

Issue Six: This relates to the myth of the dividing line between good people and those who do evil, possessing the "violent seed" that, as another demon of the theocratic conception of the Middle Ages, resides within them (Stone 2009).[2] The complexity and diversity of evil does not allow for a comprehensive and satisfactory response. As a consequence of extreme, incomprehensible violence being enshrined in history, in modern times, especially in our all the more secular era, the feeling of an insufficient development of its content has arisen.

The above fact was accompanied, unfortunately, by the hesitation of psychoanalytic thinking to focus on describing it and, therefore, dealing with it. In support of the above evaluative "unfortunately" I mentioned, I would like to quote the relevant words of the father of Psychology of the Self, Heinz Kohut, whose important help in understanding violence has been overlooked:

So long as we turn away from these phenomena in terror and disgust and indignantly declare them to be a reversal to barbarism, a regression to the primitive and animal-like, so long do we deprive ourselves of the chance of increasing our understanding of human aggressivity and our master over it.

(Kohut 1972, 378)

"However, the truth is – it must be admitted with sadness – that such events are not bestial, in the primary sense of the word, but that they are decidedly human" (Kohut 1972, 378). Accepting the limits of human understanding of phenomena as complex and primary as evil in man, I think it is good to remember even in such difficult mental conditions as those that extreme violence causes us, that psychoanalysis has already broadened people's perception in relation to the unconscious or preconscious level of mental life of all of us – both as perpetrators and as victims.

J. Rose has reflected on this and mentions the following themes from works by authors from regions of the world where violence against women is prevalent – such as South Africa – underlining that at any rate, the need to recognize deeper desires within each hero is a central theme of the books: a young woman who has suffered sexual violence discovers that she was somehow looking for the violence that destroyed her; someone else realized that she had within her own desire for bloody violence, that she was getting a deep pleasure from it. All these stories overturn the original perception of the victim (Rose 2021, 32).

Let no one rush and be disturbed that women are thus accused of seeking the violence to which they are subjected. Vulnerability to violence, for example, through inadequate protection, is the symptom and cannot legitimately be capsized as the cause of violence. After all, the theme of the seduction of evil is central to the study of violence. Do we deal so much with violence because of the seduction it causes us (the media is flooded with it, as are the tv series and books) and, on the other hand, we seek the quick, conscious renunciation of violence within us in all its expressions because of the intolerable and nuclear existence of evil within the psyche of us all?

Issue Seven: The Search for the Root of Violence: Is the abuse of the abuser in childhood responsible? (Jacquot et al. 2018). As Michael Stone concludes after extensive study, in his book *The Anatomy of Evil*, there is no single profile or a biography that fits all cases of violent behavior (Stone 2009, p. 200). In other words, although there is clearly too often an element of a traumatic childhood, it is neither a necessary nor a sufficient condition for becoming violent. Stone presents many cases and gradations of violent behavior, but very few cases of people who were abused and did not become violent themselves – as he points out, their names are not left in our memory.

Sometimes, as for example in the case of Aziz that I will present, her own violence comes as a reaction to the escalation of violence she suffered and her inability to respond in a way that she feels fair within the culture in which she suffered the trauma of rape. As the root of violence, reference is often made (and rightly so, in my opinion) to a previous narcissistic wound that seeks reparation through revenge in every way, both on an individual level and on a collective level. But what constitutes a narcissistic wound?

In his *New Introductory Lectures on Psycho-Analysis* (1933, 66), Freud referred to the writer Emil Ludwig (without naming him) and his fictional biography of Emperor Wilhelm II (1926) based on Alfred Adler's thesis on the inferiority of organs (Adler 1907). Ludwig interpreted the Emperor's tendency to be offended and turn to war, as a reaction to a particular sense of inferiority of the organs. The Emperor was born with one hand atrophied. The defective limb became the wound that remained open throughout his life and was expressed in the specific character formation which, according to Ludwig, was one of the major factors leading to the outbreak of World War I. Freud disagreed with the above interpretation and argued that it was not the congenital problem per se that resulted in Emperor William's susceptibility to narcissistic insults, but the rejection by his proud mother, who could not tolerate a child who was not perfect (Kohut 1972). The introduction of narcissism was a crucial point in the thought of Freud (1914), and its forms and transformations were particularly explored by Heinz Kohut (1966). The latter particularly studied the feeling of shame that follows a narcissistic blow and paves the way for narcissistic rage in an attempt at revenge and the desire for magical reparation (1972).

Issue Eight: Does psychoanalysis have anything to offer to the extent that neither truly evil nor highly abused people ever reach its "couch"? I tried to answer this question regarding the potential of psychoanalysis to help with the refugee issue (Giannoulaki 2023; Christopoulou et al. 2023). Having presented the topics, we will start in the same way as psychoanalysis, from case study, taking particular account of countertransference (in other words, from the psychoanalytic method of research to psychoanalysis).

Clinical Material

Aziz does not come from a poor background, nor does she come from the most violent countries in Africa. She is a young woman from Tunisia. Tunisia is the North African country where the "Arab Spring" began and the only democracy that emerged from this uprising. Despite the constant crises in its political life, there have also been reforms that attempt to reduce the power of the religion of Islam and the separation of the state from the umma (Saegesser 2023). I cite elements from religion, society, and family structure because they are necessary to better understand and control countertransference in meeting a person from a different cultural environment (Nadig 2023). Refugees to Lesvos come from many diverse cultures and countries, mainly from Asia and Africa.

Returning to Aziz: She was referred to a psychologist for banging her head on the floor and threatening to kill herself. She cried constantly and, in addition, created serious quarrels with the other refugees in the camp. The psychologist did not understand what she was saying, although he was always assisted by an interpreter. He wondered if Aziz suffered thought disorder and underwent a melancholic, psychotic, delirium. The question of diagnosis and appropriate treatment made her one of the six refugees who asked for my psychiatric assessment.

Aziz came with her head covered by a headscarf, looking down, visibly angry. Aziz spoke in Arabic but in a rare dialect, as the interpreter informed me. Unable to translate Aziz's speech in a flowing way, he repeatedly asked my permission to interrupt her and ask her what she meant. While Aziz initially spoke coherently, as the interpreter asked her repeatedly to help him by writing down on paper the word he was having difficulty translating, gradually her speech became rambling. The interpreter could not form a coherent speech. He communicated unrelated talk, the content of which gave the impression of delirium. For example, Aziz would say something like, "For my sake, her husband divorced my sister. It is my fault!" I wondered if this referred to a real incident of an incestuous affair with her sister's husband that led to the couple's separation. Was it an incestuous wish that came true or a fantasy against the sister?

Aziz's emotion moved between loud crying and anger, and progressively, escalated in intensity. The interpreter was ready to cry as Aziz yelled at him and seemed ready to attack him; I was in a state of increasing wonder and sense of helplessness, when fortunately, I heard among her cries a word that I recognized as French. The word "complètement" which means "completely," After clarifying that she knows French well, which I happened to know too, it was possible for her to tell me the following:

A fortnight before her wedding in Tunisia, she was raped by someone in the wider group of friends of her future partner. Rape in her culture, imposed her abandonment by her future husband, because she was now no longer "pure", and her marriage to the rapist to cleanse her family. When her future husband refused to leave her (they have come to Moria together), the need for catharsis was transferred and the sister's husband took over to divorce the sister, as a representative of Aziz, as this man was distantly related to Aziz's partner. Aziz and her partner were now social pariahs and were hiding, while the rapist not only did not hide, being respectable since he declared that he intended to marry her but was also entitled to send her angry messages claiming her. One day, two years after the rape, her rapist once again messaged her, "When I tell you to come somewhere, you will come and do what I tell you," setting again a meeting point. While usually Aziz simply did not pay attention to his messages, that day, blind with despair and rage, she went to the meeting point and threw so much vitriol at his face and body that she almost killed him.

Listening carefully to this account, without the intervention of an interpreter, in French, I can confess that I was drawn into an identification with her, fervently desiring revenge on the rapist. "Well done to him! He deserved this, even death for all the suffering he had caused her!" Accustomed to questioning my emotional reactions, countertransference, especially if it is too intense, I retreated with difficulty, trying to control the cheerful fantasy that Aziz was able to defeat him. Curiously, I was reminded of the novel *Beloved* (Morrison 1989) and what followed the joy when Seth managed to escape.[3] Did my feelings make me so careless? Did I become part of a mob, adopting as a just punishment the method of lynching, used in cultures against women who do not obey the Kuran? An eye for an eye... Mitigating with the above mental process the inebriation that had initially seized me, I sufficed to tell her that it took bravery, perseverance, and patience to survive mentally in the circumstances of the rape and what followed.

Aziz seems to have taken the self-esteem bracing "nourishment" I gave her – the reflection of a humane, understandable in desperation, reaction – and proudly said:

> I have my partner who loves me very much! He's here with me! We are gone together! Every time I get caught up in crises, he holds my hands, so I don't hurt myself. When the rape came out, because I had to have an operation on my genital area because of the destruction of my body, he tried to say that he raped me. But they didn't believe him and didn't let him marry me. He supports me and tells me when I want to kill myself, that I am a good woman, that I am a scientist, and I do not deserve to beat myself up! My parents don't understand me, they don't forgive me! This is done in Arab countries! As soon as this happened, I stopped leaving the house, stayed in a room, and stared into the void. I went to a psychiatrist, and he gave me medication, my sister hid me. The rapist wouldn't leave me alone though! This is why I went and threw acid in his face. That's why we left!"

She is sobbing, then continues: "I want my life back! I found myself here in a tent in Moria and having nothing."

I told her that I understood that her threatened ruin through a marriage to the rapist was so unthinkable that it led to the act of violence that forced her to leave her country and find herself in Moria (with little prospect of getting a residence permit in Europe as she was not one of those who fled a war zone, something I thought about but chose not to mention at this point). Aziz seemed to feel my attempt to understand what happened to her. She thanked me, still crying. At the end, she took off her headscarf, showing her well-groomed and dyed hair with highlights, and greeted me with a handshake. Did I have in front of me the lawyer that she was before the rape? I certainly did not have in front of me the woman who asked me if she was psychotic.

Elements of Theory

Being raped once as an adult is perhaps the mildest form of violence one can hear in Moria camp where there are hundreds of women who are victims of incest, gang rape, and subsequent forced marriage to one of the rapists. Marriage is the only way out if they do not want to be murdered by a male member of the paternal family – to cleanse the shame of the family after the rape. In Moria, as in Athens where I worked as a supervisor in hosting structures for women who were victims of violence, I met many who lived and had children with their rapist, forced to endure their rape daily, seeing no end to their abuse and paradoxically not "desiring" to help them get out of this situation. Unlike most refugees, before her rape, Aziz is educated, works as a lawyer with a particularly good salary, owns a house and car in Tunisia, loves her future husband, and he loves her too. All of the above do not make her a woman who can easily succumb to a life of constant abuse.

The relationship between culture and violence is an inexhaustible field of thought and research (Freud 1930) that we cannot delve into further in this work. The lack of empathy in her environment (for example, her parents refused to meet and listen to her since) constantly increased the violence she had suffered over time and continued to suffer from her religion and culture. There came a critical moment in Aziz's life when she heard her parents pressuring her older sister to refuse housing to her so she would be forced to accept marriage to the rapist and put an end to this peculiar condition of voluntary isolation that seemed unable to end otherwise. Her sister offered her the only refuge and if she sent her away, she would have to agree to marry her rapist. Aziz could not allow this to happen, as she emphatically told me. Whether she would be killed, or kill was nothing compared to the threatened degrading of her personality, if she was forced to follow the rapist. Her mood is reminiscent of the heroine of *Beloved*, which came to mind. The interpreter's inability to understand what Aziz was saying on a literal level served as a goad to the metaphorical inability to understand what was happening to her by other people within the general cultural context of her homeland.

Meanwhile, in cultures such as hers, the rapist bases his masculinity on acquiring the "woman," and this can help to understand (not tolerate or forgive) why the rapist of Aziz claimed his "plunder" by saying everywhere that Aziz is *his*, his property and will not allow her to marry another or return to work (De Vincenzo and Troisi 2018). Culture allowed the rapist, like the slave traders of *Beloved,* the attitude of claiming or even imposing it on him so that he could feel like a respectable member of society.

When it comes to acid revenge, I think it is important to think that many times, hidden behind an impulsive, violent act, there is a ritual desire to repair the wound: as if there was any chance that Aziz would regain her face and her life if she destroyed the face and life of the abuser. This desire remained naturally unconscious for Aziz. The act of violence often has primordial symbolism (Ricoeur 1967) that the abuser cannot put into words. If Aziz had gone to a psychoanalyst instead of a psychiatrist, she might have avoided the violence of the acid attack, which further stigmatized her life. Possibly not. Perhaps, the devastation caused by the rape would not allow reparation for this particular woman. I do not have that much evidence to arrive at such an opinion.

Returning to the meeting with her, I think that the mitigation of my own violence and the enjoyment of a violent attitude, even under the guise of doing justice, without going to the other extreme of its condemnation, contributed to showing in her response both: the pride in her uprising and the realistic acknowledgment that because of it she is in Moria, in aggravated conditions. Realistically, it was an act of revenge that escalated the violence against Aziz, putting her at risk of years of imprisonment (with consequent exposure to the multifaceted and continuous violence of prisons) and the need to take the road of exile. I think the desire to lynch the rapist gave way to the desire to give voice to Aziz and what her own act of "revenge violence" attempted to express. Even so, Aziz wanted to talk to me. On my next visit to the camp, she waited for me and greeted me with a smile.

I possibly want to give voice to her story also because of the guilt that I could not go further with her in the given circumstances, beyond this one meeting and the relevant instructions to the psychologist and the team of caregivers of Médecins du Monde. After the meeting, I was thinking about how the inability to treat one as human being, the lack of interest in one's feelings and thoughts, even if one cannot express them in words because of the trauma they have suffered, creates the pinnacle of violence: the murder of the psyche, reminiscent of Judge Schreber and his delirium.

The goal of therapy, argues psychoanalyst Caroline Garland writing of Ms. O, who was also a rape victim, is to turn the "impossible for man's mind to grasp" into something that the victim of violence can think about and keep in their mind without fleeing (Garland 1998, 110). Garland emphasizes that it seems easy to say but exceedingly difficult to achieve this goal with victims of violence and terror, as many patients are.

In this chapter, I acknowledge that I asked many questions, possibly more than the space of a book chapter allows to unfold. The answer to questions, such as those concerning extreme violence, evil in Man, is beyond not only the potential of a text, but also human understanding in general; nonetheless, I believe that thinking about all levels of violence facilitates delving in aspects of it – a delving that can in turn help understand and prevent some of its expressions. For example, addressing violence against women through the adoption of a stereotypically masculine, energetic attitude – a punitive attitude in the name of a moral and intellectual superiority – is a defense that psychoanalysis can illuminate, thus preventing the escalation of violence.

Psychoanalysis has as its constant aim the vigilance at the danger of alignment with current views, prejudices, racism that seduce toward the abandonment of psychoanalytic radicalism. Indeed, I think the desire to prioritize thought is radical. Violence breeds violence and the public's demand for "just" punishment of the guilty in any area, vengeful violence encouraged by the media, is dangerous. The ferocious demand for the violent annihilation of Evil by placing it outside us reassures our Superego, lulling to sleep the internal, controlling authority as a search for justice.

Therefore, the limitation of violence must start from the limitation of violence within us, as I have tried to show that I achieved, partly through the decision to abandon the feeling of triumph ("She served him right!"). Abandoning my sense of narcissistic, unrealistic triumph allowed me to feel both regret and guilt for what I could not offer and for the best position I was in – and despair and a sense of liability for Aziz's ongoing turmoil. The sense of responsibility partly led me to give voice to Aziz through this text, highlighting the intercultural dimension of the phenomenon and hoping to give a helping hand in the arduous task of caregivers of victims of violence and caregivers of perpetrators, refugees, or others.

Notes

1 (a) Changing laws to facilitate divorce. (b) Special centers where abused women and their children can find shelter (1,200 centers in the United States at the time Gilligan wrote his book served over 300,000 women and children, enabling them to leave the abusive husband and take their children with them). (c) Social awareness of women's rights. (d) Changing moral attitudes toward what constitutes unacceptable and abusive behavior. (e) Offer of work and income so that abused women can leave the abusive partner, and so on.
2 Although we cannot exclude the possibility of the existence of a hereditary burden, therefore a "wild seed" (Stone 2009, 320).
3 After a joyous celebration for Seth and her children, when they are discovered by the traffickers to drive them back into slavery, no one seems willing to help by notifying Seth in time. Blind with rage, Seth kills her 2-year-old daughter, Beloved, with a saw. The plot is based on a true story.

Bibliography

Adler, Alfred. 1917. *Study of Organ Inferiority and Its Psychical Compensation*. New York: Nervous Mental Disease Publishing Co. Originally published 1907.

Atwood, E., and Robert D. Stolorow. 1993. *Faces in a Cloud: Intersubjectivity in Personality Theory*. London and New York: Jason Aronson Books.

Christopoulou, A., C. Giannoulaki, and N. Tzavaras. 2023. "Mourning and Identity Issues in the Treatment of Refugees in Lesvos." In *Trauma, Flight, and Migration: Psychoanalytic Perspectives*, edited by the series IPA in the Community. London and New York: Routledge.

Cooke, Jo. 2022. "Call This Violence What It Is." *New York Times*, December 28. Opinion, Guest Essay.

Giannoulaki, Chrysi. 2020. *Heinz Kohut: Narcissism and Psychoanalysis*. Athens: Indiktos Publications.

Giannoulaki, Chrysi. 2023. "Is Psychoanalysis of Any Help for Refugees?" In *Trauma, Flight, and Migration: Psychoanalytic Perspectives*, edited by the series IPA in the Community, London and New York: Routledge.

De Vincenzo, M., and G. Troisi. 2018. "Jusqu'à ce que la mort nous sépare: Silence and Alienation dans les Violences Conjugales." *Topique: La Psychanalyse Aujourd'hui* 143 (2): 111–24.

Freud, Sigmund. 1911. "The Case of Schreber." In *The Standard Edition of the Complete Psychological Works of Sigmund Freud*, edited and translated by James Strachey, vol. 12, 3–85. London: The Hogarth Press.

Freud, Sigmund. 1914. "On Narcissism: An Introduction." In *The Standard Edition of the Complete Psychological Works of Sigmund Freud*, edited and translated by James Strachey, vol. 14, 67–102. London: The Hogarth Press.

Freud, Sigmund. 1930. "Civilization and Its Discontents." In *The Standard Edition of the Complete Psychological Works of Sigmund Freud*, edited and translated by James Strachey, vol. 21, 57–146. London: The Hogarth Press.

Freud, Sigmund. 1933. "New Introductory Lectures on Psychoanalysis." In *The Standard Edition of the Complete Psychological Works of Sigmund Freud*, edited and translated by James Strachey, vol. 22, 3–182. London: The Hogarth Press.

Freud, Sigmund. 1937. "Analysis Terminable and Interminable." In *The Standard Edition of the Complete Psychological Works of Sigmund Freud*, edited and translated by James Strachey, vol. 23, 209–54. London: The Hogarth Press.

Gammeltoft, Tina M. 2016. "Silence as a Response to Everyday Violence: Understanding Domination and Distress Through the Lens of Fantasy." *Ethos* 44 (4): 427–47.

Garland, Caroline. 1998. *Understanding Trauma: A Psychoanalytical Approach*. London and New York: Karnac Books.

Gilligan, James. 1997. *Violence: Reflections on a National Epidemic*. New York: Vintage Books.

Jacquot, M., A. Thevenot, M. P. Chevalerias, and C. Metz. 2018. "Violences Conjugales: L'énigme du Lien aux Racines de l'Infantile." *Topique: La Psychanalyse Aujourd'hui* 143 (2): 99–110.

Kohut, Heinz. 1966. "Forms and Metamorphoses of Narcissism." *Journal of the American Psychoanalytic Association* 14: 243–72.

Kohut, Heinz. 1972. "Thoughts on Narcissism and Narcissistic Rage." *Psychoanalytic Study of the Child* 27: 360–400.

Kohut, Heinz. 1982. "Introspection, Empathy, and the Semi-Circle of Mental Health." *International Journal of Psychoanalysis* 63: 395–407.

Laufer, L., and T. Ayouch. 2018. "Violences Conjugales, Famille, Vulnérabilité (Domestic Abuse, Family, Vulnerability): A Psychoanalytical Approach." *Topique: La Psychanalyse Aujourd'hui* 143 (2): 151–67.

Leuzinger-Bohleber, Marianne, G. Schlesinger-Kipe, and N. Hettich. 2023. "What Has Clinical Psychoanalysis to Offer to Traumatized Refugees? Some Experiences During the So-Called 'Refugee Crisis' in Hesse (Germany): Part I: The STEP-BY-STEP Project, Part II: Psychoanalytic Treatments of Refugees in Kassel." In *Trauma, Flight, and Migration: Psychoanalytic Perspectives*, edited in the series IPA in the Community, London and New York: Routledge.

Ludwig, Emil. 1926. *Kaiser Wilhelm II*. Translated by M. Colburn. London and New York: Putnam.

Masson, Jeffrey. 1985. *The Complete Letters of Sigmund Freud to Wilhelm Fliess.* Cambridge, MA, and London: Belknap Press of Harvard University Press.

Morrison, Toni. 1989. *Beloved.* Translated into Greek by Elli Kallifatidi. Athens: Cloud. Originally published 1987.

Nadig, M. 2023. "Trauma, Refugees, and Ethnopsychoanalytical Experiences." In *Trauma, Flight, and Migration: Psychoanalytic Perspectives*, edited by the series IPA in the Community. London and New York: Routledge.

Petrucelli, J. 2018. "Introduction: Can We Live and Work Securely in Our Bodies? It Is Time to Talk." *Contemporary Psychoanalysis* 54 (4): 621–33.

Ricoeur, Paul. 1967. *The Symbolism of Evil.* Translated by Emerson Buchanan. New York: Harper and Row.

Rose, Jacqueline. 2021. *On Violence and on Violence Against Women.* New York: Farrar, Straus, and Giroux.

Saegesser, B. 2023. "Fifteen Years of Psychoanalytical Fieldwork in Eastern African Cities." In *Trauma, Flight, and Migration: Psychoanalytic Perspectives*, edited by the series IPA in the Community, London and New York: Routledge.

Snider, N. 2018. "'Why Didn't She Walk Away?' Silence, Complicity, and the Subtle Force of Toxic Femininity." *Contemporary Psychoanalysis* 54 (4): 763–77.

Stein, Arlene. 2014. *Cupid's Knife: Women's Anger and Agency in Violent Relationships. Part of Psychoanalysis in a New Key Book Series.* New York and London: Routledge.

Stone, Michael. 2009. *The Anatomy of Evil.* USA: Prometheus Books.

5   Identity and Mourning

The Question

Refugees are, by definition, faced with multiple griefs: mourning for the place and life they left behind, often irreversibly, mourning for loved ones who died in disasters, mourning for parts of themselves that they will not find again, such as their health damaged by torture and amputations, their social, economic, or professional position, and more.

Refugees are simultaneously facing a less obvious but significant identity crisis due to:

(a) Mourning processes where "the shadows of objects fall on the ego" (Freud 1917), breaking the core of their identity through the invasion of "ghosts" that the psyche is unable to "assimilate" or "kill."
(b) The need to adapt to the host country by adapting their identity accordingly.

A new element added to the sense of self of the refugees is that each of them, regardless of whom they have been back in their country of origin, is now someone whose present and future depend on the asylum service and its judgment. An affirmative answer to his asylum application will allow him to have a residence and work permit. At that point, he will be able to leave the closed refugee camps and/or seek his fortune by moving freely in the country, in this case to continental Greece and through it to the EU. Therefore, the asylum interview process is a daily discussion in Moria, and elsewhere with refugee accommodation structures in Lesvos, because doctors' and psychologists' offices are swarmed by refugees seeking certificates that would facilitate their receiving of the much-desired asylum. The members of the committees at the asylum-seeking interview examine the request, considering the accompanying certificates. The regulations based on which the right to asylum is granted are far from clear and firm.

The relevant scene in Finnish director Aki Kaurismäki's film *The Other Side of Hope* (2017) about a Syrian migrant, Khaled, seeking asylum in Finland, in Helsinki, where he has arrived and lives in a dormitory with other refugees, is characteristically tragicomic. In this scene, the decision refusal of

DOI: 10.4324/9781003639022-6

the Finnish state to grant asylum to the Syrian refugee is announced in a serious tone. In Aleppo (where the protagonist has already lost his home, parents, and little brother to a missile), they say to him, "conditions do not pose a threat to all residents, so the applicant is not entitled to asylum and must be repatriated." Alongside the announcement of the unfavorable decision, the viewer watches on a television screen image from Aleppo, where buildings are demolished by missiles and children are taken injured to a hospital.

Even though NGOs prevent their employees from being involved in assessing asylum applications, this is practically impossible because the conditions allow for loopholes where each caregiver can exceptionally decide to help a particular refugee. Moral conflict is inevitable since the weight of a "no" (in other words, "I will not help you escape an unjust and imponderable law that probably leads you to death") is also great and has grave consequences for the particular subject. On the other hand, there is also great moral conflict regarding the inability of any caregiver to have the ability to say "yes" to all requests for help as legislation and the particular laws of the country do not allow it.

In Kaurismäki's film, after the adverse decision opens the door for his deportation the next day, an employee opens the back door, allowing Khaled to escape (thus allowing him to later reunite with his sister, who arrives in Finland via another dangerous refugee route). From this point on, the film's main plot begins, which focuses on the interaction of Khaled and a Finn; Wikstrom, who gradually abandons his wife, quits his job, earns money in poker, and buys a restaurant. After their first quarrel, a friendship is formed that will "save" them, each from their dead end. As *New York Times* critic A.O. Scott (Nov. 30/2017) writes, Finnish writer and director Kaurismäki "is less a satirical observer of his nation's foibles than an excavator of its mopey, mordant, steadfast conscience" (Scott 2017).

Similar to Wikstrom, who at first is annoyed by Khaled sleeping next to the garbage outside his restaurant, refugee caregivers who undertake rapid and unpredictable treatments in charged conditions (survival needs, acute bereavement, asylum claim, fear of repatriation, difficulty communicating due to different languages) face some degree of disruption of their therapeutic identity by the mass influx of the *Stranger* into their familiar therapeutic but also more generally cultural, religious, and geographical area, stirring within them phenomena of racism and xenophobia. Refugees are not credible because they want to elicit the coveted certificate, so they lie by exaggerating any symptom in order to succeed in being classified as belonging to the "vulnerable" about whom a decision to repatriate or return to the country from which they entered the EU (in this case Turkey) will put their health and lives at risk of death.

Because of the importance of the above situation, refugees will do anything to obtain favorable treatment and often arrive prepared by other refugees for how to behave in order to obtain a document that will facilitate the asylum process. As an Iranian immigrant advises the Syrian in Kaurismäki's film: "It helps to smile because the melancholic ones are sent back more easily, but do not smile on the street because they will mistake you for crazy."

In order to facilitate the psychic experience of the annoyance and anger that caused Wikström not to tolerate Khaled in the first place, we can refer to literature and Marcel Proust at the beginning of *In Search of Time Lost* and hear how he described something similar – nonetheless of much less intensity:

> It is however, unspeakable the discomfort caused to me by this inva-
> sion of mystery and beauty in a chamber that I had finally managed
> to fill with my ego so much that I did not pay more attention to it than
> to my ego. As soon as the anesthetic effect of habit ended, I began to
> feel things so sad.
>
> (Proust 1997, 19)

Although the writer is simply talking about the invasion of a magic lantern in his room at bedtime (or perhaps precisely because he is talking about something so seemingly simple), he manages to capture extremely clearly the discomfort from the invasion of the strange element into the intimate space.

The biographical sense of continuity that goes unnoticed in normal circumstances is disturbed when excitation is too great for the psyche to flow in from the outside world. Then, various psychic processes take place to allow the return to what is familiar by confronting the disturbing strange element that has poured in and altered the existing psychic reality.

Through the understanding that literary description facilitates, we "step into each other's shoes" and are prepared for the defense mechanisms that occupy all of us in order to confront with clarity the racism and xenophobia that stir within us and that can take on many facets. An important and often recurring aspect of invisible and pitiful racism is the rejection not perhaps of the refugee himself – who could quickly be condemned by conscience – but of what he carries with him, for example, his diversity.

Rejection can consist of denying the cultural reality of the other (which is why the intercultural approach is a tool of significant importance in the refugee crisis) and refuting his mental reality. If the above refutation occurs and pity and charity remain, our therapeutic identity is lost as we lose the way to listen under the narratives of what is happening in the psyche. What remains is an attitude disguised as humanism that turns refugees collectively into victims, along with a desire to offer practical goods, which, however helpful, quickly wears off – and the therapist along with it.

The very effect of trauma on refugees makes them powerless to benefit from aid when it is not given appropriately: for example, by considering their culture, their habits, and plans for their future (in the formation of which they should be helped if they do not already exist), or their preparation for asylum denial and repatriation. Refuge care's central goal is facilitating the grieving process with particular attention to identity resistance. How can we process the grief (acute or chronic) of the refugee, his ambivalence that accompanies Oedipal conflicts, and his narcissistic battles to gain his self-esteem, avoiding listening only with the ear of pity to the accounts of his suffering?

In refugee camps, we are often confronted with the fact that the refugee often resists the prompts and/or wishes of the therapist, for example, for a woman to learn English and Greek so that she can work and ask for a divorce from the rapist who became her husband, and they had children together. As a result of identity resistance, for example, the refugee may become pregnant again, and the therapist may feel helpless and a sense of frustration that will cause him to give up his therapeutic work. Identity resistance is well-known in psychoanalytic literature, although it is not often mentioned. Thomä and Kächele consider identity phenomenologically as the Siamese twin of the self (Thomä and Kächele 1987, 135). Typically, one is internally possessed by a sense of undisturbed continuity that procures one with the firm conviction that one is oneself without much question about what one perceives as one's identity (Erikson 1956).

In Erikson's thought, identity is the regulator of an important resistance stemming from the need to protect it:

Identity resistance is a universal form of resistance that is always experienced but not often recognized during analyses. It is the patient's fear that the analyst, because of his particular personality, his influences, his philosophy, can intentionally or unintentionally destroy the weak core of the patient's identity and impose on him his own. The therapist must patiently prove that he can maintain understanding and care for the patient in repeated crises without devouring him or offering himself for a totemic meal.

(Erikson 1956, 214–15)

Erikson's protection of identity alludes to the importance of Kohut's sense of self, and both can be subsumed under Freud's *Principle of Self-Preservation*, from which resistances and defenses begin, especially in the first period of his thought. In psychoanalytic theory and clinical work, it has been repeatedly emphasized that the various defense functions of the psychic apparatus serve, among other things, the Principle of Maintaining Safety, which is often more important than pleasure/displeasure or else the Pleasure Principle (Sandler 1960).

In some cases, such as the case of Luigi, a 30-year-old young man who was helped by humanitarian organizations to leave Congo, where his life was in danger because of his human rights work, it was easier to mobilize the health practitioner to overcome her own resistance and understand how to facilitate his adaptation to the conditions of Lesvos while he was waiting for the help promised by the UNHCR (United Nations High Commissioner for Refugees).[1]

Luigi is one of those whom Eisold calls "heroes," highlighting the self-lessness with which they have fought for human rights in particularly dangerous circumstances. Despite their resilience, moral stature, and intelligence, the author observed that their adaptation to the United States has not been as successful as their previous resistance activity (Eisold 2019). How can we think in order to be better prepared to understand them and contribute to their adaptation to the new conditions?

Clinical Material

From the first session, where Luigi came to seek help with his insomnia and the physical pains that tormented him, he spoke clearly about his loneliness and frustration with the asylum service process:

> They told me to wait. They promised that it would be easy to get asy-lum because of my activism in Congo. I was disappointed again and again. I pressed my lawyer, called him, and rather annoyed him, but he never called me back. Therefore, I am on my own. I want to get out of here, too; maybe it is better to be alone. Alone, like in prison where no one can visit you and help you.

Luigi suffered more from loneliness and frustration than from his physical pains, for which he had initially turned to the facility's medical services.

His family had converted to Catholicism and practiced their religion with devotion to Africa. He had a human rights activism that put his life at risk, mainly inspired by his father's actions. He was not just a refugee who fled his country for his life, but someone who left only after all his relatives and friends, and especially his father, pressured him to do so because, at his subsequent arrest, he was bound to be killed. Luigi spoke about his loved ones killed by rival political organizations, his arrests, and the abuse he had suffered in prison (stabbing in various parts of the body, electric shocks under torture, etc.). Luigi showed his wounds, saying neither his words nor his fingers were enough to count the number of times he had been taken to hospital after arrests. With each new imprisonment, Luigi (who witnessed the rape and murder of fellow inmates) thought only of revenge. With each new release from prison, Luigi, as a devout Catholic, tried to find a way to forgive his torturers – as Christ teaches, he added. Because of his activism and the torture he had been subjected to repeatedly, Luigi received special assistance. He was transferred out of the closed camp of Moria to a shelter on Lesvos, where he was offered psychodynamic therapy at a rate of once a week that lasted for several months. It should be noted that Luigi's treatment is something that few refugees have access to before relocating to large urban centers.

After several sessions and while the therapist had partially gained his trust, Luigi spoke of his guilt over his mother's death during a protest. His mother received a murderous knife blow; he believed his mother deliberately entered the knife trajectory to save him. Luigi's father accused him of being responsible for her death – at least that is what he believed. Then, Luigi, at his father's urging and insistence, left Congo because of the dangers to his life, and then the rest of the family members left in different and unknown directions. At present, Luigi could not communicate with his relatives for safety reasons, not even knowing if his family were alive and safe somewhere or imprisoned or even dead.

Luigi came late to his sessions but managed to talk about his sense of being trapped in the shelter in a way that made the therapist do her best to help him: "I'm scared. Winter is here. I feel trapped again in a prison. Prison got me the taste for life. I lost everything: the feeling of being alive! I feel like an animal!" The practitioner noticed that each time his religious feeling came to his aid. He added, for example: "If there were no suffering and sorrow, there would be no priests who offer comfort to the faithful and no saints."

With the help of supervision, the therapist thought of relying on his character trait to act in favor of others and suggested to him, after consultation with the camp's management, to become more involved in the lives of other refugees, which pleased him greatly. In a subsequent session, he said, "I feel like I am helping. Every time they listen to me, it is like a gift from God." Of course, Luigi, in this way, was as if he took on a caregiver function that exposed him to similar problems, as his African fellow citizens soon did not content themselves with his speeches and supportive words but complained to him about where to sleep, about food that was not good and other practical matters.

In one session, Luigi spoke of his fatigue and frustration, saying that he felt he had to withdraw somehow but, at the same time, also thought that this would be incompatible with the activist's identity. Then, respecting again his identity and ideals, his therapist, knowingly resorting to a slight manic simile, claimed that it is normal for him to want to rest since God Himself, after creating the world, on the seventh day, wanted to rest. Luigi's gaze changed immediately, and he remained silent. As the session drew to a close, the practitioner added that there were still 2 minutes left. This remark forcibly brought him back to reality, so he reacted with these words: "I would like to say that the only precious thing I have to offer the world is time. ... For me, being a revolutionary means turning negative people into positive ones and not limiting yourself to your status quo." The reminder of time served as a counterweight to the manic dimension of comparison with God and allowed Luigi to regain a down-to-earth self-confidence. His identity as a religious activist was an important element that supported him. His role and identity allowed him to borrow people of identification from religion. For example, he identified with Abraham as a refugee, observing that Abraham had also left his homeland.

Elements of Theory

The psychodynamic approach is considered appropriate for a significant number of severely injured people, and they even prefer it themselves in the midst of other therapies offered, for example trauma-focused therapies (van der Kolk et al. 1996).

This is because in cases of extreme post-traumatic stress disorder (PTSD), there are areas of personality that are not easy to improve with trauma-oriented therapies. On the contrary, psychoanalysis, with its attention to agitation due to the trauma of older, internalized relationships with the object, and the deepening of the defensive processes that any loss entails, can potentially offer better support in the post-trauma period to the sufferer in various areas of his personality. Such areas are, for example, the need to strengthen self-esteem and self-formation, the need to weaken the defensive reactions of the psyche as a consequence of trauma through the reinforcement of self-observation and speech (in other words, the strengthening of symbolic function at the expense of the one-dimensional, timeless domination of specific discourse – concreteness and lack of dimensionality), the need to internalize safe ways of relating to the other (where basic trust in the other has collapsed), the need to improve the integration of the extremely traumatized person into relationship networks (where usually the rupture of the family and social fabric has contributed to flight). These are therapeutic goals for which psychoanalytic thinking has much to offer (Schottenbauer et al. 2008).

As I have already written, Luigi's case belongs to the category of "heroes" among asylum seekers from different regions of the world that Barbara Eisold presents in her book *Psychodynamic Perspectives on Asylum Seekers and the Asylum-Seeking Process* (2019). Indeed, as Eisold observes on a number of occasions, Luigi was the eldest son who, with his intelligence and moral stature, undertook to embody the sacred ideals of his family, resisting persecution and torture at the risk of his life. The author explores what allowed each of the 11 "heroes" asylum seekers in the United States to abandon their role as a dissident fighter in their own country. In Luigi's case, I think it was the survivor's guilt that led him to a move that was partly self-defeating for him. Although fleeing his country leads him to salvation, experiencing the simultaneous paternal exhortation to leave as punishment for his mother's death shows his deep guilt for having survived while his mother died.

If this deep guilt is not addressed, Luigi will not be able to benefit from the help offered to him and will wander from camp to camp and country to country as "a wild and solitary animal," as he has described himself. It is not only prison and persecution that made him lose his sense of being alive, but the guilt that in an instant he saw his beloved mother fall next to him dead, without him being able to react and save her.

The research already conducted by psychoanalysts on the victims of the Holocaust has created concepts such as the *survivor syndrome*, very useful for understanding and therefore treating the severely traumatized people of our time. For example, W.G. Niederland, in his article "Clinical Observations on the Survivor's Syndrome," looking for the consequences of the extreme trauma suffered by 800 survivors of Nazi persecution – many survivors of concentration camps – found that they suffered from chronic depressive states, which covered the entire spectrum: from masochistic character changes to psychotic depression. He linked the severity of depressive states to "guilt of the survivor" (Niederland 1968; 1981).

The guilt of the survivor is considered very important. The Norwegian psychoanalyst Sverve Varvin, who has been particularly involved in treatment methods in cases of extreme trauma (Varvin 2003), argues that "one must remember that what makes survivors suffer unimaginably is that they have witnessed others who have been killed or tortured without being able to help or protect them" (Varvin 2003, 74). He adds that the survivor's guilt that had been somewhat forgotten after studies of Holocaust survivors re-surfaced in Norway after the July 22, 2011, terrorist attacks on the island of Utoya that killed 77 people. The survivors' *guilt* weighed heavily on the young people who survived (Varvin 2003). In surveys, one in four Norwegians was affected by these unexpected attacks in a country like theirs.

In survivor syndrome, beneficial points have been described for understanding the effect of extreme trauma on the psyche: points that without this knowledge can lead to fragmented and panicked reactions of those who undertake the treatment of these people, symmetrical to the fragmentation that the psyche undergoes during trauma. For example, the many physical pains, the phenomena of disconnection, and the psychotic manifestations pose continuous diagnostic issues that must, of course, be examined individually but also within the overall clinical picture of the survivor's syndrome. The typical triad of symptoms of the survivor is considered by Niederland (1968) to be the following: migraines, persistent nightmares, and chronic depression followed by various psychosomatic symptoms.

A model of survivor syndrome is traumatic neurosis or war neurosis – a process generally described as a continuous revival of the unconscious conflicts caused by the traumatic situation. Lately, more importance has been given to the representation of the loss/death caused by trauma more than the trauma itself. A symptom of great importance, and not only phenomenologically, is the transformation of victims from trauma that can be attributed to the image that they experience themselves but also appear to others as if they are living dead; in other words, as if they live in an intermediate space between the living and the dead. They are no longer alive as they were before the trauma occurred; they have not died like other companions in the trauma space, but they cannot get out of this intermediate space-time. They are like ghosts that evoke something ineffable in others but leave a unique aroma in the whole personality (Lifton 1973; 1976).

In the line of thought of Freud, where the deepening into an extreme mental condition is treated as the starting point to understand analogous situations of milder intensity and shorter duration that the everyday person faces in normal conditions of life, R.J. Lifton, American psychiatrist, studying the psychology of the survivor stated:

> I see this process in terms of the psychology of the survivor as I have elaborated that psychology in my work on Hiroshima and more recently with antiwar veterans. My belief is that survivor conflicts emerge from and apply to everyday psychological experience as well. When one outlives something or someone, and there are of course many large and small survivals in anyone's life, the specter of premature death becomes vivid. Simultaneously one begins to feel what I came to call "guilt over survival priority": the notion that one's life was purchased at the cost of another's; that one was able to survive because someone else died. This is a classical survivor process and is very much involved in traumatic neurosis.
>
> (Lifton 1973, 11)

Lifton writes:

> Death anxiety can be seen as a signal or threat to the organism, a threat now understood as disintegration, stasis or separation. All anxiety relates to these equivalents of death imagery, and guilt too is generated insofar as one makes oneself "responsible" for these processes.
>
> (Lifton 1973, 10)

Lifton distinguishes between a static (either numbed or self-lacerating) and an animating guilt. He considers the latter important for the process of self-transformation. The therapist, with the help of the supervision, tried to move Luigi's guilt from static to one that brings to life, relying on the identity of the religious activist. I believe that if the therapist's psychodynamic understanding of the root of the problem was not considered, there could only be a demand to adapt to the present situation, thus a further loss of identity and a burden on the grieving process with which Luigi was confronted.

A great number of writers, such as Wilhelm Steckel, Otto Rank, and others, have described patterns that closely resemble this psychic numbing as the essence of neurosis. Steckel in 1908 spoke of neurotics who "die every day" and "who play the game of death" (Stekel 1973, 131). Otto Rank also refers to a continuous restriction of life, because someone "refuses the loan (life) in order to avoid the payment of the debt (death)" (Lifton 1973, 11).

Clinically, there seems to be a strong connection to unresolved and complicated grief and sadness, and beneath self-blame are often repressed anger and resentment against those who have been lost (e.g., parents) for failing to protect patients from persecution. The survivor takes as persecution what happened to them from their salvation onward. Possibly, Luigi holds his father responsible, and through the defense of projection, he feels that his father rejects him as responsible. Besides, the father's attitude that pushes him to flee to save himself reinforces the above position.

The practitioner and the supervisor sought the place where the battle against the Furies, against the demons of Luigi, could be fought: a sacred space. In Luigi's case, this space is his encounter with the God of Christians and Abraham of the Old Testament through his identity as a religious activist. Davoine and Gaudilliere cite another example of a sacred ground from Pat Barker's trilogy that I have already mentioned, which resembles Dr Rivers's identity as a researcher in the Solomon Islands:

> On the last page of the trilogy, Njiru, Rivers's informant in the Solomon Islands, appears to him in the middle of London, in the military hospital, coming to the rescue when he, the doctor, has to face so many young people dying and killed in battle.
>
> (Davoine and Gaudilliere, 306 in French, 323 in the
> Greek transl.)

The two psychoanalysts link the psychoanalytic function in this case to the term "ritual man" created by Wittgenstein to approach these necessary places and practices in times of disaster (ibid, 322).

Note

1 The historical dimension of the principle of reality does not forget Marcuse's observation in this regard: "The principle of reality supports the human organism in the external world, which in the case of man, is a historical world. The external world, which the developing ego faces at every stage, is a socio-historical organization" (Marcuse, Eros and Civilization, 34). In the context of the historical dimension of the principle of reality, it is important to know that in September 2016, world leaders met at the United Nations to adopt the New York Declaration for Refugees and Migrants, a document in which many nations committed themselves to the protection of migrants and refugees in a host of different ways. Despite this declaration, the willingness of potential host countries declines every day sharply.

Bibliography

Davoine, Françoise, and Jean-Max Gaudillière. 2004. *History Beyond Trauma*. New York: Other Press. Originally published in French as *Histoire et trauma: La folie des guerres*. Paris: Stock, 2006.

Eisold, Bernard K. 2019. *Psychodynamic Perspectives on Asylum Seekers and the Asylum-Seeking Process: Encountering Well-Founded Fear*. London: Routledge.

Erikson, Erik H. 1956. "The Problem of Ego Identity." *Journal of the American Psychoanalytic Association* 4: 56–121.

Erikson, Erik H. 1968. *Identity, Youth, and Crisis*. New York: Norton.

Freud, Sigmund. 1917. "Mourning and Melancholia." In *The Standard Edition of the Complete Psychological Works of Sigmund Freud*, edited and translated by James Strachey, vol. 14, 237–58. London: The Hogarth Press.

Kohut, Heinz. 1971. *The Analysis of the Self*. New York: University Press.

Lifton, Robert J. 1973. "The Sense of Immortality: On Death and the Continuity of Life." *American Journal of Psychoanalysis* 33 (1): 3–15.

Lifton, Robert J. 1976. *The Life of the Self*. New York: Simon.

Marcuse, Herbert. 1955. *Eros and Civilization*. Boston: Beacon Press.

Niederland, William G. 1968. "Clinical Observations on the 'Survivor Syndrome.'" *International Journal of Psychoanalysis* 49: 313–15.

Niederland, William G. 1981. "The Survivor Syndrome: Further Observations and Dimensions." *Journal of the American Psychoanalytic Association* 29: 413–25.

Proust, Marcel. 1997. *À la Recherche du Temps Perdu*. Translated by P. Zanna as *In Search of Lost Time*. Athens: French Institute at Athens, 1997.

Rank, Otto. 1958. *Beyond Psychology*. New York: Dover Reprint.

Sandler, Joseph. 1960. "The Background of Safety." *International Journal of Psychoanalysis* 41: 352–56.

Schottenbauer, Michele A., Carol R. Glass, Diane B. Arnkoff, and Sara H. Gray. 2008. "Contributions of Psychodynamic Approaches to Treatment of PTSD and Trauma: A Review of the Empirical Treatment and Psychopathology Literature." *Psychiatry* 71 (1): 13–34.

Siegel, Mark A. 1996. *Heinz Kohut and the Psychology of the Self*. London and New York: Routledge.

Scott, A. O. 2017. "Review: In The Other Side of Hope, an Old-Fashioned Humanist Fable." *New York Times*, November 30. NYT Critics' Pick.

Stekel, Wilhelm. 1964. *Nervous Anxiety States and Their Treatment*. Translated by Rosalie Gabler. New York: Dodd Mead and Co. Originally published in 1923. Cited in Jacques Choron, *Modern Man and Mortality*. New York: Macmillan, 1973.

Tzavaras, Nikos. 2002. *Hermeneutics and Understanding in Schizophrenia: A Phenomenological and Psychoanalytic Approach*. Athens: Kastaniotis Publications.

The Other Side of Hope. 2017. Directed and written by Aki Kaurismäki.

Thomä, Helmut, and Horst Kächele. 1987. *Psychoanalytic Practice: Volume 1 – Principles*. Berlin: Springer-Verlag.

Van der Kolk, Bessel. 2014. *The Body Keeps the Score: Mind, Brain, and Body in the Transformation of Trauma*. London: Allen Lane.

Van der Kolk, Bessel A., Alexander C. McFarlane, and Lars Weisaeth. 1996. *Traumatic Stress*. New York: Guilford Press.

Van Essen, John. 1999. "The Capacity to Live Alone: Unaccompanied Refugee Minors in the Netherlands." *Mind and Human Interaction* 10: 26–34.

Varvin, Sverre. 2003. *Mental Survival Strategies After Extreme Traumatisation*. Copenhagen: Multivers.

Varvin, Sverre. 2016. "Psychoanalysis with the Traumatized Patient: Helping to Survive Extreme Experiences and Complicated Loss." *International Forum of Psychoanalysis* 25 (2): 73–80.

Volkan, Vamik D. 2017. *Immigrants and Refugees: Trauma, Perennial Mourning, Prejudice, and Border Psychology.* London: Karnac Books.

6 Forms of Repetition

The Question

Since 2016, when I went to Lesvos, I have worked in the refugee field in one way or another – perhaps because I need to metabolize what I experienced (and still experience) in my work with refugees and their caregivers. In the text *Is Psychoanalysis of Any Help for Refugees* (Giannoulaki 2023), I described an experience that was short but considerable in internal tension, which I was particularly concerned about. I referred to it often to understand later clinical experiences (as I will show in this chapter), and I quote it below:

> On Sundays, when I go to the camp to see the refugee patients, the children play in front of the door, which keeps the place guarded. Unaccompanied minors are kept in containers also in a guarded area outside and in front of the first reception area where the clinics are located. One Sunday, going out in a hurry to catch the plane back to Athens, I found the door closed, and outside, six or seven children were five to eight years old. Energized from their game, they have tied the door on their side with a cord and look at me defiantly, shouting, "No good I.D.! No good I.D.!" For seconds, I do not understand what is going on, and I feel a shiver of terror disproportionate to both my position and my age in front of this small mob of Lilliputian guards who "imprison" me in the camp, closing the door with a toy string.
> Meanwhile, a guard intervenes, and the door opens. I caught the plane. Even if it came from children, even if it is a game, the voices "I.D. no good! No good ID!" the voices echo in my memory for the next few days, and I remember the sparks of rage in the eyes of the little refugees along with the excitement of joy of children's play.
> (Giannoulaki 2023)

I often worked on cases of unaccompanied minors in caregivers' support groups, as they are always a source of problems and concern in the camp and shelters for the unaccompanied children in Athens. I had not been in direct contact with them. As I am not a child psychiatrist, the caregivers did not send me requests for their diagnosis and treatment. In the

DOI: 10.4324/9781003639022-7

original text (2023), I wrote that I automatically resorted within myself to the well-known *game For-Da* of Freud's grandson that transported me to another place, the place of thought and removed me from the space of the Lilliputian violence.

As I think about it in retrospect, writing this book, I think I froze in terror in front of the closed door. Only after the intervention of the guard, ashamed of my terror and the sense of the ridiculousness that accompanied it inside me, did I turn to my psychoanalytic identity to lean on and feel my narcissistic balance return. In a way, I created a *cover story* that hid the moment I was ashamed of by constructing something that gave me identity and healed the rift in my self-esteem. What kind of phenomenon was it that I was confronted with this Sunday when the cute little children, who at other times I liked to see playing in the yard allotted to them, turned into a terrifying mob? I can only understand my horror as theirs that found in this way, through play, the means to express itself. Understanding the other means through empathy, I can reliably represent his experience corresponding to one of my own. The experience I have as a psychoanalyst in meeting the analysand at a given moment, my countertransference is a point of attraction for my attention, especially when it is the source of a sense of uncanny that forces me to process the overall state of my psyche.

It has been described by people dealing with refugees the sudden appearance of something – a sentence, a movement, an image – that comes as a message from the past that has not been symbolized in search of a psyche that can metabolize it, give it psychic content. Once this "creation" appears – in the above case a game – it can be internalized by a psychic apparatus that, to the extent that it can bear it, will attempt to understand it in psychic terms. The above mental work is not easy.

Virginia Micco (2019) refers to the immense fatigue required by conversion work

> that permeates the flesh and psyche ... for anyone who will offer to welcome, even for a while, these psychic fragments that have caused the psychic uprooting. ... Contact with anyone who bears within them the traces of traumatic uprooting leaves no one untouched. It continues to create an endless uprooting to anyone who approaches.
>
> (Micco 2019, 29)

Psychoanalysts who have dealt with trauma have described how the person who has experienced a catastrophic event – an event that therefore exceeds his mental endurance and makes him feel helpless and completely powerless – enters a vortex of regression that sucks him toward the stage of his life before words, before the conquest of symbolic thought (Garland 1998).

By playing, children actively repeat something they have experienced passively and obviously traumatically during the refugee period and continue to experience it in the camp. In trauma we have something that repeats itself in an automated way. But how is it repeated? Does the subject perceive repetition? Does it cause him discomfort, or is it some repetition that is in tune with his ego? Does it belong to his biography in a way that does not alienate him, or is it the entrance of a foreign element that breaks the identity of the subject? When an analyst is suddenly confronted with the fragments of someone's wounded psyche where he is unable to discern a narrative, a certain coherence, a point where associations seem to converge into meaning, the introspection of these fragments tends to mobilize his own destructiveness. The easy target is the injured people themselves, the objects of care. However, the above introjection can also become the starting point for understanding what happens to the refugee.

Donald Moss, the guest speaker at the 16th Annual Conference of the Hellenic Psychoanalytic Society on *Evil*, spoke about it. I will quote the relevant excerpt from the interview he gave me for the psychoanalytic journal *Oedipus*:

> There is a kind of internal representation of evil where one is under constant threat from a force that declares that one's existence is illegitimate, that one is not welcome here, that one has no place here. At any time, he can be thrown out, he can be banished. I think that the above condition is not an unusual internal state of the psyche, and we can identify the dynamics of Evil in it. I think sometimes analysts are frightened and don't respect the depth of this internal logic of extermination. They say something like, "You hate yourself. You feel guilty. You want to punish yourself." I think these forms of representation are reassuring to the analyst because they are much milder than what I am trying to say right now. This is not a punishment; it is not guilt. It is something much more elementary than that, more basic. In this condition the individual lives constantly with this sense of insecurity, of uncertainty as to whether he has the right to exist. It is a completely different interpretation from "You feel guilty."
>
> (Moss 2025)

believe that the experience I had in the seconds of the game was in the order of the logic of extermination and helped me understand the clinical material from the expulsion of a "difficult" teenager from a facility for unaccompanied adolescents in Athens. "Difficult" are called the refugees who, through the continuous violation of the rules of operation of the camp and self-injurious behavior, push the caregivers and other co-habitants in the camp to no longer be able to deal with them and want to "throw them out." In these relatively frequent cases in refugee camps for unaccompanied children, someone becomes the scapegoat, one who ceases to meet the criteria of "a person who needs help" and becomes the "person who disrupts the structure, and we must kick him out." I think these are the cases we need additional tools to understand.

Only with the help of colleagues to whom I refer in this book, of texts and discussions, can I accept, for example, that my shame after the incident with the game in Moria was not only because I was scared, but mainly because I momentarily hated children. For a brief moment, I was furious with anger toward them and wanted to get them out of the way because I could not wait to get to the airport. Through *my* horror, I knew not only *how* terrified the children were, but also *how* terrified those who approached them became. Through my destructiveness that I managed to recognize within myself, I knew how destructive a caregiver can be in such situations. In particular, at the institutional level, where compliance with the rules can conceal hatred and divert attention from suffering one manifests in an untreated and brutal, therefore violent, way, the ability to recognize hatred in caregivers needs to be highlighted.

Clinical Material

In one of the supervisions of a group of caregivers in a shelter for unaccompanied teenage refugees, I unexpectedly and surprisingly found myself in an atmosphere of hilarity and relief. The caregivers exchanged jokes and recounted how they had spent the day before. As this feast was not frequent in an admittedly difficult situation, such as working in this facility, I felt awkward, almost unfamiliar. I felt outside the group, as I could not share their feeling, and, slightly annoyed, I thought that a manic connotation characterized the dominant feeling.

Soon, there was greater calm, and then I was informed that they had "finally" managed to evict a 14-year-old teenager from the facility who was creating constant problems with his disobedience to the rules and regulations there. I had heard about this teenager in previous supervisions as well as the constant efforts of caregivers to evict him, which is not institutionally easy when it comes to an underage guest. We had already talked about the many traumatic losses of this teenager. I also remembered that this boy had lost his therapist at the facility when she recently took childbirth and postpartum leave.

Kadan, the expelled teenager, had experienced being evicted from his family in Syria as a punitive decision by his father. I did not have much biographical information about this teenager. However, I knew that often parents send their most capable children along with other fellow citizens on the refugee journey, thinking that it will offer them a better life. Unfortunately, children are often not adequately prepared for this decision, resulting in fantasies of Oedipal and a murderous attitude from the respective parent. The ensuing reactions of anger and destruction are expected consequences if they are not softened by someone who will take it upon themselves to be a surrogate parent into adulthood. I tried to steer the new therapist in this direction in a previous supervision. So, obviously, Kadan's expulsion from the camp triggered a sense of failure for me to help him and the team members. I got angry with the caregivers, and my anger was noticed even though I thought I was hiding it. A therapist looked at me defiantly and said she was not interested in any refugee as long as she could return home safe and sound at night. I was bitten in an attempt to control my anger over what I considered to be a blatantly destructive decision.

Kadan did not do anything extremely destructive. He poured salt on the caregiver's coffee and threatened the previous pregnant therapist with hitting her baby, but he did not. On the other hand, Kadan threatened other teenagers in the camp when they did not do what he asked, for example, to watch a particular show on TV, and the caregivers suspected that there was also sexual abuse of younger teenagers by him. However, whatever Kadan's behavioral problems, I felt that the realistic assessment of the hosting structure's failure, the accompanying guilt, the mourning for the therapeutic (and human) relationship that had been destroyed, had been covered under a cloak of hilarity and sympathy among those present, which was impossible not only to empathize with but also to tolerate. They behaved as if they had won over a sadistic, common enemy. Only the enemy was one of the teenagers they had taken care of. They arrived to the point of saying that Kadan was happier now that he had managed to leave the camp and that they could see him wandering outside smiling.

The interpreter came in late; he was of the same nationality as the expelled teenager and spoke the same language, and he spoke about the teenager's despair, his loneliness, the dangers he ran at this sensitive age living in an open, unprotected facility for adults where he had been transferred. He said Kadan would come every evening across the street from the camp looking to feel safe at the only place where he had been last received. He had already been exploited by drug dealers who wanted to use him as a drug courier. As the interpreter spoke, I felt my ability to think return, and my aggression decreased. The interpreter acted like the man who opened the door to Moria. My turn toward the memory of what I had experienced in Moria, Lesvos, when the unaccompanied refugee children, kids in the latency period, momentarily took on the dimension of sadistic torturers came to my mind. The sadistic torturers were now the caregivers themselves. My momentary despair in Moria in the seconds I waited for someone to rescue me and open the door helped me understand the desperation of the group members who were waiting for someone to open the door and free themselves from their tormentor, the teenager who had for his reasons been trapped in repeating the behavior that caused his expulsion.

Once I realized the pervasive destructiveness of which I was becoming a tool, I said nothing "psychoanalytical" for the rest of the session, for example, a psychoanalytic interpretation of what happened. My goal became to be able to leave the group in an atmosphere of calm, unstimulated, reconnection with each other, an atmosphere of diminishing anxiety about the present and future of each member, as expressed by the young woman who said she just wanted to return home safely. I left thinking that the goal of a good functioning of the institution for the reception of unaccompanied minor refugees always remains one of the most difficult issues in the refugee field.

Elements of Theory

It is documented that it may be impossible for traumatized persons, all the more so children and adolescents, to create a coherent narrative about their traumatic experiences. So, their ability to communicate their experiences is feeble and sometimes even impossible, depending on their age and capacity for symbolization and verbal expression.

We know, as psychoanalysts, that children communicate through playing. However, after severe trauma, the play takes on the form of a repetitive scene, like the game in Moria (a reenactment) or the provocative behavior of Kadan, who attempts to attract attention by terrorizing the caregivers (an enactment). There are descriptions in cases of severely traumatized children, of PTSD symptoms in the surviving family members that become triggered by the play or the acting out of the child (Junod, Sidiropoulou, and Schechter 2022). I believe that something analogous happened to me and the members of the caregivers' group of Kadan. The so-called "side-effect" of post-traumatic play can impair the caregivers' emotional availability and ability to connect intersubjectively with the child or the adolescent.

Rephrased the question in this chapter is as follows: can the process of our own response to the violence of refugees, here unaccompanied minors, prevent or minimize the problem? Can psychoanalytic theory and clinical psychoanalytic thinking offer tools for the integration and tolerance of the extremely traumatized individual, and especially minors in networks of relationships, when often the rupture of the family and social web has contributed to the flight, as here probably to the expulsion of Kadan from Syria? (Schottenbauer et al. 2008).

In a traditional psychoanalytical way of seeing, the analyst understands the other person through empathy. He is not part of the relational system of two individuals – such as a mother–child dyad – but he tries to function as a "third" who keeps in mind the other's verbal and nonverbal elements, here the traumatic experience. It is a fact that a subject can have a reliable representation of someone else's feelings, desires, fantasies, and more generally of someone else's inner world because of a particular ability of man which is considered to belong to his basic endowment. However, this ability has great limitations, especially in marginal areas of injured people, restrictions with catastrophic consequences if they are not recognized as such.

Although I know the opinion that follows as expressed in a personal conversation, a young psychologist, regarding her hesitation to begin her psychoanalytic training, claimed that she feared that the intended formation of a psychoanalytic identity would prevent her from spontaneously relating to the suffering person. The therapist stands firmly in the therapeutic tradition, professing that it is good to be reticent of partial and erroneous human knowledge. In his book *The Body Does Not Forget*, Bessel Van Der Kolk refers to his teacher, Elvin Semrad, who taught him to be skeptical of psychiatry textbooks. He said, "We had only one real textbook: our patients. We should trust only what we could learn from them – and our experience" (Van Der Kolk 2014, 11). However, Van Der Kolk says that Semrad himself said: "even as he pushed us to rely upon self-knowledge, he also warned us how difficult that process is since human beings are experts in wishful thinking and obscuring the truth" (ibid). Especially in adolescent hosting structures, phenomena of resonance of their own pathology of boundaries and challenging behavior are created due to the pathological disconnection of bonds within the institution and the creation of conflicts between caregivers that lead to the failure of support and psychosocial rehabilitation of "difficult" adolescents. It is also well documented that the caregivers run the risk of being traumatized because of the work with the traumatized people.

Michel De M' Uzan refers to Theodor Reik (1937), who pointed out that listening to the patient requires the analyst to observe his ego or, more precisely, a part of his ego that is transformed by taking the object into himself. "One could even say that at certain extreme moments of the process, the analyst becomes the patient" (M. de M' Uzan 2013, p 101).

The great hostility that caregivers create toward the unaccompanied refugee minor is, in my opinion, a rupture, a regression of the group caused by the tremendous preverbal violence of infanticide Kadan experienced because of his expatriation from his family.

The great hostility that exists from the child toward the mother and even more so from the mother toward the child and primarily toward the son was a point of constant denial by Freud. George Atwood and Robert Stolorow, in a book considered the starting point of the intersubjective approach, titled *Faces in the Cloud* (1993), chose to proceed with a psychobiographical analysis of four authors of psychological theories (Freud, Jung, Reich, and Rank) in an attempt to highlight the influence of specific elements of their biography on their theory. The authors highlight the effect of Freud's constant defensive function on the need to save his relationship with his mother from any hostility. The son's relationship with the mother becomes an object to be fully defended. As late as 1930, he wrote in *Civilization and Its Discontents*: Aggression ... forms the basis of any relationship of affection and love in humans (with the sole exception, perhaps, of the mother's relationship with her male child) (Freud 1930, 113).

Oedipus Rex, who completes the incestuous relations of the Labdacidae myth, is complemented in the dimension of infanticide by another tragedy, the Bacchae, which highlights the dark part of the cult of Dionysus. The patricide of Oedipus has left in the shadow the attempt at infanticide of

Laius, to Jocasta's knowledge. Claudio Laks Eizirik at the Delphi conference on the subject of the Father said that in the field of mythology it is
recorded in different traditions that patriarchal societies in order to exist
and expand are based on dysfunctional father–son relationships, which
prove that the process of separation and differentiation from a frightening gigantic paternal figure is carried out in a relentless and extreme way
(Bazaridis 2023, 41). However, Stavroula Berati wrote that infanticide has
been largely ignored in psychoanalytic literature and adds that this may
be because infanticide is much more frightening for most of us and easily
covered by the shadow of denial[1] (Beratis 2022, 116). In Euripides' *Bacchae*,
it emerges that Dionysus does not dwell on laurel-crowned epic and lyric
poets and, of course, does not dwell on the logical arguments of Socrates.
He "dwells" in the horrors of cannibalism, in terror in the face of the chaos
of the human soul, and in the attempt of collective oblivion of the unimaginable evil that one man does to another, even if it is one's son, as is the
case with Agave and Pentheus. Perhaps, I became the cruel superego and
its sadistic attitude toward the group members. The "holes," the deficits, in
the psyche of traumatized minors create the "holes" in the way the caregivers work, which in turn allows repeated destructive acting out.

The ordinary man has a sense of identity and a constant, for the most
part, collection of memories and ways of behaving that characterize him as
a person. This is the autobiographical self (Damasio 1999). In my opinion,
the disturbing experience in front of the game in Moria and the maniacal
feast of the team in Athens shocked me because they led me to feel the Evil
within me, the destructiveness within me. Getting out of what you think
is yourself, getting out of the familiar, to find the deepest core of yourself, the familiar that is scary, the tragic inside you, is always a disturbing
experience.

Traumatic events are impossible to put into words, at first. On the one
hand, if we insist to speak prematurely about the trauma, the patient's preoccupation with trauma can only be strengthened and fixated on it. On the
other hand, silence can lead to mental death.

How will the words be found to talk about what one cannot enunciate?
We need the inner process, the translation of the disconnected side of our
own self into words that will create a bridge with the rest of the self; and
then, the above connection will act as a core catalyst for the connection
of the disconnected bonds of self and group, individual and institution.
Therefore, we have to pay attention to accommodating not only adolescents in the hosting facility but the intolerable dissociated parts of their self
and their experiences within the psyche.

This is often an impossible job. As Michel de M' Uzan puts it: "The analysand is felt to be someone who may become an intruder whom an analyst
in difficulty would attack within himself in a similar manner to the way
in which he may be attacked." I attacked the caregivers as they attacked
Kadan. They attacked Kadan as he attacked the caregivers, enacting his

trauma. All that is needed is that the above mental activities be gathered and used toward an interest in understanding and possibly helping the children in Moria, Kadan in Athens, and their caregivers regain their human identity.

The recognition of the human dimension of the other and, therefore, of our Self passes through the recognition of the particularity and suffering that he carries inward and deposits within us. The loss of an empathetic and understanding environment creates the anxiety of disorganization, which is the most serious of all anxieties. The loss of the empathetic environment leads to disorganization because it entails the loss of satisfaction with the most basic human need, which is to be treated as an individual with a psychological existence and a psychic world. The need to be respected as a person with a psyche is like the air we breathe; we cannot live without it.

In order to outline the importance of the empathetic human environment, which is essential to human psychological existence and is lost when evil prevails, Kohut mentions the following incident:

> A spacecraft was hit by a meteorite before landing on the moon. The control center on Earth asks the astronauts what they prefer since they have lost control of the spacecraft: to leave the craft free to orbit the moon or to pull it back to Earth, but because of the damage, they will not be able to control its speed and, therefore, it was very likely that due to friction they would be charred. The astronauts did not hesitate to choose to return to Earth (although eventually, the damage was repaired, and they returned safe and sound). As they say, it was unbearable to think they would wander forever in a non-human environment. They said the Earth is our home, even if we return charred.
>
> (Kohut 1981, 531)

Finding again the capacity to think after such an attack to links gets someone stronger and in a way more human. Nietzsche's intuitive perception of the discontinuity of the sense of self led to the emergence of Dionysus as Apollo's rival awe in order to access what is ineffable and frightening. I will quote some of Nietzsche's relevant words:

> The drama did not start just because someone disguised himself and went to fool a few others, but rather because he was "outside of himself" and believed that he had magically been transformed in the state of the "being outside of himself," of ecstasy. We need only go one step further: we do not return to ourselves, but we put on another existence ... in the final analysis, this is where the profound surprise of drama as a spectacle comes from: the ground trembles, faith in the inseparability and solidity of the individual is shaken.
>
> (Nietzsche 1870 in 2009, 12)

Note

1 But the cruel superego and its sadistic attitude toward the ego, especially in melancholy, may be a way through which infanticidal desires find a way of expression. After all, the superego is the representation of our introjected parents, and the ego largely retains children's parts in all of us.

Bibliography

Atwood, G. E. and Stolorow, R. D. (1993). Faces in a Cloud. Intersubjectivity in Personality Theory. Jason Aronson. Rowman & Littlefield Publishers, INC.

Bazaridis, Kostas. 2023. "Talking about the Father." In *The Father: Psychoanalytic Perspectives*, edited by Luigi Zoja. Athens: Armos Publications.

Berati S. (2022). Commentary in Jacqueline Amati-Mehler' s paper Fatherwood's Destinies. In *Father. Psychoanalytic Perspectives*, edited by Bazaridis, K. and Hatziandreou, M. Athens: Armos books.

Beratis, Stavroula. 2023. "Comment on J. Amati-Mehler's Paper: The Destinies of Fatherhood." In *The Father: Psychoanalytic Perspectives*, edited by Luigi Zoja. Athens: Armos Publications.

Damasio, Antonio. 1999. *Le Sentiment Même de Soi*. Translated by C. Larsonneur and C. Tiercelin. Paris: Odile Jacob.

DeM'Uzan, Michel. 2013. "During the Session: Considerations on the Analyst's Mental Functioning (1989)." In *Death and Identity: Being and the Psycho-Sexual Drama*, edited by Michel DeM'Uzan. London: Karnac, 2013. New York: Routledge, 2010.

Freud, Sigmund. 1930. "Civilization and Its Discontents." In *The Standard Edition of the Complete Psychological Works of Sigmund Freud*, edited by James Strachey, vol. 21, 64–145. London: Hogarth Press, 1953.

Garland, Caroline. 1998. "Issues in Treatment: A Case of Rape." In *Understanding Trauma: A Psychoanalytic Approach*, edited by Caroline Garland. London and New York: Karnac.

Giannoulaki, Chrysi. 2023. "Is Psychoanalysis of Any Help for Refugees?" In *Trauma, Flight and Migration: Psychoanalytic Perspectives*, edited by IPA in the Community. London and New York: Routledge.

Giannoulaki, C and Moss, D. (2025). Interview with Donald Moss Oedipus, edited by Armos, vol. 28.

Junod, Nicolas, Olga Sidiropoulou, and David N. Schechter. 2022. "Case Report: Psychotherapy of a 10-Year-Old Afghani Refugee with Post-Traumatic Stress Disorder and Dissociative Absences." *Frontiers in Psychiatry* 13: 940862. https://doi.org/10.3389/fpsyt.2022.940862

Kohut, Heinz. 1981. "On Empathy." In *The Search for the Self: Selected Writings of Heinz Kohut: 1978–1981*, vol. IV, edited by Paul Ornstein, 531. Karnac, UK, 2011.

Levine, H. B. 2009. "Time and Timelessness: Inscription and Representation." *Journal of the American Psychoanalytic Association* 57: 333–55.

LaFarge, Louise. 2014. "On Time and Deepening in Psychoanalysis." *Psychoanalytic Dialogues* 24: 304–16.

Micco, Vincenzo. 2019. "Esprits Migrants, Esprits Adolescents: Transitions, Transformations, Migrations: Avancer sur les Marges." *Revue Belge de Psychanalyse* 15: 29–47.

Nietzsche, Friedrich. 1870. "The Ancient Greek Musical Drama." In *Dionysus Against a Crucifix: Essays and Notebooks (1869–1873)*, translated by Vangelis Douvaleris. Athens: Ed. Mast, 2009.

Reik, T. (1937). *Surprise and the psychoanalyst*. London: Kegal Paul, Trench & Trubner.

Scarfone, Donald. 2006. "A Matter of Time: Actual Time and the Production of the Past." *Psychoanalytic Quarterly* 75: 807–34.

Schottenbauer, M. A., C. R. Glass, D. B. Arnkoff, and S. H. Gray. 2008. "Contributions of Psychodynamic Approaches to Treatment of PTSD and Trauma: A Review of the Empirical Treatment and Psychopathology Literature." *Psychiatry* 71(1): 13–34.

Stolorow, Robert, and George Atwood. 1979. *Faces in a Cloud*. Northvale: Aronson.

Van der Kolk, Bessel. *The Body Keeps the Score: Brain, Mind and Body in the Healing of Trauma*. New York: Viking, 2014.

7 "Difficult" Refugees and Sex Work

The Question

In the first part of the book, I referred to working with refugees in Lesvos, trying to highlight the conditions and issues where refugees are first received as soon as they leave the boats in Greek territory.

In the second part of the book, I refer to the movement of refugees to the capital of Greece, Athens. There, refugees live in specially designed camps in the city or on the outskirts or in rented apartments or hotel rooms.

In the second part of their journey, refugees' entry into accommodation structures and support from advocacy agencies and refugee communities highlight even more the difficulties in the integration of the refugees in everyday life in the host country. Many refugees or asylum seekers describe their conditions after arrival, even in more affluent countries, as the worst part of their refugee journey – without access to health care, poor sanitation, insufficient food, and minimal human concern. On a daily basis, they face inactivity, and the possibility of being forced to return to their homelands. This is described by many as mental torture (Varvin 2019).

What happens during the settlement period in accommodation structures and while waiting for the answer from the asylum services – which can take years – is of decisive importance for the present and future integration of the refugee into the social network of the host country, for their mental health and their quality of life, especially for vulnerable refugees such as unaccompanied minors: mothers with young children, patients (whether they were mentally and/or physically ill before leaving their country of origin or fell ill on the way), the elderly, and those who have been victims of torture and/or mutilation.

Due to their major and complex problems, refugees highlight the shortcomings in the host countries' health and welfare systems. For example, in Lesvos, understaffing in the psychiatric clinic makes it impossible to treat a psychiatric patient who needs involuntary hospitalization. However, the shortage is covered by the possibility of transferring the patient to Athens or Thessaloniki. However, when the refugee has no right to move, the court order for involuntary hospitalization highlights the problem. However, on

DOI: 10.4324/9781003639022-8

the other hand, it can be the "solution" for the refugees leaving the island, as happened in the case of Bahar, which I will present in this chapter.

On mainland Greece, it is easier to find a way to flee and (illegally) travel to other countries in Europe, which are the final destination of many of the refugees. From the island, this movement is much more difficult. The desire to flee is so strong that even a parent can abandon the burden and responsibilities of caring for the most vulnerable family members by leaving alone for another country in Europe, with the excuse of later bringing the rest of the family with them. For example, in Athens, where a psychologist visited a refugee family to help integrate children into the school system, the interpreter translated a note from the father for her two weeks later. The father said he thanked her for taking over his family and could now leave for Germany, where his brother had already settled.

In general, families face a variety of crises: a member is ill and needs special care, and/or a member suffers from PTSD and has outbursts of anger or resorts to alcohol or substances and more. All the above may lead to the breakdown of the family. Often, the collapse of the family requires an urgent intervention of the social services of the housing structure, such as when parents or the mother stop sending the family's children to school, or when a family member commits suicide, or when episodes of abuse of the wife or children by the husband are reported.

In Athens, the program EPAPSY (Association for Regional Development and Mental Health) was created with the aim to try to respond to the need to support refugees in this phase of their journey (during their arrival from the islands to Athens and Thessaloniki) in parallel with international bodies promoting the integration of refugees in this transitional stage as well as with UNHCR. EPAPSY has been providing mental health services to refugees and asylum seekers with severe psychosocial difficulties since March 2018 through a mobile unit. The aim was to have a liaison function between the different refugee care services to fill the gap in their coordination, something that proved particularly difficult in many cases where the deficits of the host state, in the case of EPAPSY, Greece, may not have the corresponding services, for example, to help an autistic adolescent who presents outbursts of aggression in the family.

The above example is not accidental, as it has repeatedly concerned us. For example, in a refugee family with an autistic teenager, the older brother committed suicide under the burden of the responsibility of caring for her and moving her to health services that her parents were unable to undertake. In another case of an autistic teenager, during the visit of the EPAPSY psychologist with the interpreter at home, there was a love attack by the 15-year-old autistic teenager on the interpreter, who was terrified and did not want to continue working with us. It should be noted that it has been impossible to find a solution to offer a daily short-term occupation for this autistic teenager with learning basic self-care activities, as this care is offered only by private centers in Athens and, again, to a limited extent.

The intervention team included a psychiatrist, a child psychiatrist, a psychologist, a social worker, and three interpreters. The particular emphasis given by this program to strengthen the bonds in the network of beneficiaries was in line with the psychodynamic understanding of each refugee individually. In the group, supervision took place by two supervisors on a regular fortnightly basis, one of whom was me. The supervision was psychodynamic.

We realized one more time that without supervision many therapeutic efforts based mainly on altruism stop when the tensions from the difficulties overflowing the psyche and body of the patient overflow the psyche and body of the caregivers too. For example, this is the case presented above, when there was an attack on a member of the group visiting difficult refugees in their place of residence. Additionally, there are tendencies of rupture in the group – expressed in the resignation of a member or the expulsion of the refugee from the camp – which, of course, is a possibility, which, nonetheless, one must carefully weigh before deciding. The difficulty of integrating the "difficult" refugee into the fabric of relations of the hosting structure is transferred to the broader society. Then, it remains more uncontrollable without the possibility of corrective interventions.

The group's goal was not only to help the refugee adapt to the very difficult conditions of his settlement but also to serve, to some extent, the path of the traumatized person toward life, closeness with others, and creation – in other words, to destabilize the effects of trauma so that they are not passed on to future generations. There have been attempts to create refugee care teams such as "Mobile teams" in Serbia organized by IAN (International Aid Network) in Belgrade, including a doctor, a nurse, a psychologist, and an interpreter, who assist refugees wherever they are, for example, parks. There has been the creation of "Michaelis Dorf" in Germany. The effort with the EPAPSY program is part of the organization of a field of thought and action. The following question is: can we help create a pool of best practices for caring for, rehabilitating, and treating individuals and families in need?

We know that the story of trauma itself is a story of ruptures. The therapeutic work with these people, the creation of bonds between the members of the group and them, the facilitation of maintaining relations between refugees and their compatriots, and the avoidance of rupture between them, as one may see in the clinical material, aims at the partial healing of the various and destructive wounds they carry on their body and psyche, even for the limited time given by the program's horizon. It has been observed beyond doubt that there is a significant potential for resilience, coping, and positive development in the refugee as a whole. It has also been argued that disaster conditions can significantly affect a person's resilience but may also bring about new abilities referred to as "Adversity Activated Development" (Papadopoulos 2007).

Clinical Material

Bahar is a young Syrian woman who made a suicide attempt in Moria and was transferred by court order to a psychiatric hospital in Athens because she could not be hospitalized in the Psychiatric Clinic in Lesvos. In addition to active suicidal ideation, there was also a general severe depressive symptomatology accompanied by multiple acts of self-harm that alarmed the hospital staff for the additional reason that they did not have an interpreter to be able to communicate with her. They asked for assistance from EPAPSY's refugee support program. Three initial meetings were held at the psychiatric hospital by the psychologist who undertook her treatment and the interpreter.

At the first meeting, Bahar was strapped to the hospital bed – the psychologist described to the group a curled-up skinny girl, battered by drugs and immobility, but with the gaze of a "wild animal" ready to attack. At the same time, however, the psychologist said she saw a beautiful young woman with tenacity and perseverance.

Although Bahar seemed to find it difficult to understand why people were interested in her, she agreed to talk about her. Bahar recounted shocking traumatic experiences such as gang rape when she was in her preteens and a marriage to one of the group, marriage that saved her from being killed to wash away the shame of rape was a turning point in her biography. The above gang rape was preceded by her work since she was a young child to contribute to the family income, where a drug addict and absent father left her mother alone to take care of many children. Bahar's story raised this time, as almost always, the question: Truth or Lie?

Is the above story true – and to what extent – or is it aimed at more favorable treatment, which amounts not only to the asylum paper or a housing apartment but also to the imaginary possibility that she will be offered all that she expects in the host country? Refugees usually expect a lot and maintain the hope that they will make it, which gives them the courage to endure such difficult conditions.

Fear of beguiling was not prevalent in the therapist, who seemed to have particularly liked her near-peer Bahar. Upon leaving the clinic, Bahar was transferred to a women's hostel in a double room with an elderly female compatriot. A small room, usually with a stuffy atmosphere from cigarettes and small cockroaches, initially prevented the psychologist and the interpreter from their weekly visit. Sessions were held in this room weekly, with the roommate waiting in the living room.

Bahar was always well-groomed, with new modern clothes, meticulous makeup, and hairstyle. At first, neighbors claimed the practitioner's attention and showed envy and rivalry with Bahar. She also experienced a narcissistic affirmation from these visits. For a few months, Bahar was strengthened. She learned to move around the city, started Greek lessons, and stopped harming himself. There were times when she demonstrated a unique ability to cope with difficulties. This ability even went so far as to treat women in a vulnerable position similar to her own. It was time to build a therapeutic alliance.

The patience with which the psychologist moved toward the suffering woman was rewarded. Bahar was empowered and built relationships with her compatriots. She met a woman who lived in a park and took her to her room, violating the rules, but at this point, the manager looked the other way. We invited the manager to the supervision team trying to create links in order to construct a human environment for Bahar. We discussed that when refugees are offered the opportunity to be active and work in the camp, they are greatly helped to form bonds with others and regain their self-esteem.

The equanimity with which the therapist moved toward the affected woman and the assistance of the whole team in the creation of a protective framework was not enough to prevent the rupture that occurred. The more Bahar was empowered, the more she was confronted with a traumatic reality. In her effort to learn the Greek language, she was confronted with the fact that volunteer teachers resigned under the weight of frustrations from this problematic population. To her request to find a job, the job search program replied that knowledge of the language is a prerequisite. At the same time, the coveted interview at the asylum service was postponed. Bahar also realized that even if she received a positive response from the asylum service, there would be a risk of exiting the accommodation program, as she would now be considered prepared enough to make her own living and able to integrate into the country.

After a few months, the problems reappeared and worsened. Bahar quarreled with the other tenants, made special demands, and injured herself whenever her demands were not met. The tensions never stopped, and the fluctuations in her mood were constant. The demands of everyday life were experienced as unbearable, the relationships with others complicated, and the financial tightness unbearable. Her hopes and expectations for the host country, like those of thousands of other refugees, were violently dashed, and she resorted to the way she had learned in her country how to cope with the tsunami of hardship.

During one session, Bahar confided in the therapist that both in her country and in Greece, she worked as a sex worker to earn the money she wanted. In that session, she was tense, cursing the interpreter and the therapist. At the same time, the social worker of the housing program received a series of complaints from residents and neighbors regarding her behavior – she brought men to the room at night after she had managed to evict the elderly roommate from it – and the violation of the institution's residence rules. That was why Bahar told her "secret" after the tenants had informed her about the protest moves against her.

Bahar confessed to her therapist that she prostitutes herself to find money for clothes and cosmetics that will make her beautiful, like Greek women. She tried to convince her that she was not a victim of trafficking. She spoke angrily to her confused therapist. Do any people prostitute her, and she hides it? Why is she afraid of them? Or why does she love them? Are they chasing her because she chose to escape from them and prostitute herself on her own? What is the truth?

It is difficult to detect the truth, especially concerning trafficking. The feelings of helplessness and hopelessness are so strong that the therapist realizes that they overwhelm her. Should she take on with someone else, an easier refugee? Is there a need for a more appropriate program for Bahar? Bahar is another difficult refugee whom everyone wants to expel because they do not know how to integrate her into the camp.

The carers involved in Bahar's treatment who made up this collaborative network (the institution's psychiatrist, psychologist, and interpreter) contacted the supervisory team. The feeling of helplessness prevailed again, as did the desire to expel Bahar from the program. She had broken all the rules and all the networks of cooperation we were building in the hope of preventing further catastrophic ruptures. Would we agree to continue with Bahar? Would they accept keeping her in the housing program?

At the next meeting, Bahar was bedridden with her foot in plaster. I quote her words as recorded by her therapist:

> He wants to kill me, and since then, I have been happy and will not denounce him (she implies something she repeats often, that her life has no meaning and better end). Last night, he came here by force into the building, and an hour before you, he came back and wanted to strangle me. My friend and neighbor stopped him. He is a relative of my husband and wants to kill me because I have humiliated them. He came here, and I wanted to leave the room and call someone to help me. As soon as I stood at the steps, he pushed me and left. I did not go out; I sat in the room, drank two glasses of alcohol, and called my friend and told her to come. As you have seen, the door at the entrance of the apartment building closes, so surely someone has given him my address, and someone has opened the door for him. No one except for the residents has keys to the door, so someone inside opened it. ... He threatens me, tells me he will kill me, and does not care if he goes to prison for fifteen years. I feel sorry for Greece because these people who threatened me in Syria come here and they get asylum. I am very sorry. Last night, if I had not left the room instead of pushing me, he could have stabbed me. No one helped me. I cried, and none of my neighbors opened their doors to come and help me. They are my compatriots; they are women like me, but no one came to help me.

She is crying.

> And in my lessons, I learned 10–15 words, but I forgot them. I'm fall-ing asleep, and I feel like I am drowning, and I scream. Since last night, as much as I have been through this far, I have remembered it all. All the mess came before my eyes. My head hurts from all the thinking that I did. ... Really, my leg, my head, and my body hurt a lot. It's better to interrupt our conversation. (Pause). ... Right now, I am having trouble speaking. I feel like I have seen everything in my sleep. I try to forget them, but I cannot.

At this point, supervision supported therapeutic stability through under-standing the function of trauma. Psychoanalysts know a lot about resist-ance. We could thus emphasize in supervision the respect for the regression that usually precedes a deepening in the relationship and the emergence of material. Just when the caregivers at the housing structure were ready to evict her, in the supervision team, we diagnosed a move forward that allowed her to become competitive with the therapist and express her anger as well as reveal her addiction to prostitution. The paralyzing effect that trauma causes by freezing the time and life of the sufferer requires a strong, persistent, and often collective effort to overcome it.

Elements of Theory

The risk of suicide is one of the significant problems in the refugee field, and the effort to prevent it is continuous and often, unfortunately, ineffec-tive. The more complex the conditions in the camps, the greater the risk of suicide. The practitioner needed to see Bahar, even when she was confined to the psychiatric hospital bed, as a young woman who wished to be beau-tiful and not just as a victim worthy of compassion. I believe that women's coquetry created as safe a space as possible between the two young women, the refugee and the psychologist, where their relationship unfolded.

In the supervision, we proposed to the therapist to make "small talk" with Bahar, trying to avoid being perceived as impinging on her. The therapist's patience and persistence at the same time reminded me of the description of creating a safe space that I had read in the case of injured children, which I shared with the team, and I will quote below:

> Through simple, rhythmic movements – herein, the therapist's ques-tions – the extent to which interaction and closeness can be tolerated is tested. The person in charge of the play program at the Trauma Center walked with a colorful ball in his hands near motionless or angry children waiting their turn in the waiting room for treatment. They did not respond to his smile. Randomly, he let the ball roll out of

his hands and approach them. When he went to collect it, he pushed it further towards the child, who initially reacted with discomfort or indifference, but gradually a smile appeared in response to the smile of the person in charge.

(Van Der Kolk 2014, 85)

A long preparatory period in which therapist and refugee establish a working alliance based on acceptance is recommended. The story of the refugee must be accepted rather than challenged. The same about the repetition compulsion. An important consequence of trauma is pleasure from pain and suffering.

After the preparatory period, there was a period of resistance and turbulence. However, it was then that the true story was exposed, at least a part of it.

After many deceptions in similar cases, where we tried in vain to "save" a refugee woman from her husband violator or sex working, we decided not to put pressure on Bahar to renounce her sex work as we thought that this was a strategy she found to deal with her many sexual traumatisms. We had to prepare her to find a better solution to earn money and feel loved and accepted. We tried to remember that her violator saved her life by accepting her plea to marry her, still not denying the violence Bahar suffered and still suffers. It was not easy for us to accept this stance as a technique to accompany Bahar, to create an empathic dyad, a shelter. According to Laub and Podell (1995), trauma implies a loss of trust in an external empathetic dyad. This results in a loss of communication with "the other" in the internal world, leading to a loss of representations and self-observing reflective capacity. So, we had in mind to help the therapist offer to Bahar this empathic dyad.

Dori Laub showed that a grave consequence of extreme traumatization is a breach in the bond to an empathic inner other (Laub 1998, 2005). This special object relation is the basis for the experience of being connected to others – and for being and feeling like a human.

Without the supervision team, the therapist would have fled from Bahar's therapy, and the manager of the shelter would have kicked her out. It would have been a disaster as the one happened with the teenager sent away from the facility. This time, we did it. I think we did it because the team's organization had aimed to care for "difficult" refugees from the beginning. In dealing with refugees where Trauma is so present, timely and appropriate treatment is of significant importance, and supervision is far from an unnecessary expense, as it is often considered.

The special feature of EPAPSY's team was caring for individual cases aiming at rehumanizing the individual, by facilitating the connection process to others and helping to reestablish essential human bonds. Being and feeling like a human is embedded in international declarations that concern human rights. Basic human rights, which include safety, the right to family, home, and protection, are integral to membership in the human community. These basic rights are given, but not stable – they have to be fought for continuously in different arenas. In this fight, psychoanalysts have their specific tasks and obligations.

(Varvin 2019)

Bibliography

Breuer, Josef, and Sigmund Freud. 2004. *Studies in Hysteria (1893–1895)*. 1893. Reprint, London: Penguin Classics.

Freud, Sigmund. 1896. "Draft K. The Neuroses of Defense (A Christmas Fairy Tale)." January 1. In *Extracts from the Fliess Papers, The Standard Edition of the Complete Psychological Works of Sigmund Freud*, edited and translated by James Strachey, vol. 1, 220–29. London: The Hogarth Press.

Freud, Sigmund. 1897. "Letter 69 (September 21)." In *Extracts from the Fliess Papers, The Standard Edition of the Complete Psychological Works of Sigmund Freud*, edited and translated by James Strachey, vol. 1, 259–61. London: The Hogarth Press.

Freud, Sigmund. 1910. "The Psycho-Analytic View of Psychogenic Disturbance of Vision." In *The Standard Edition of the Complete Psychological Works of Sigmund Freud*, edited and translated by James Strachey, vol. 11, 209–18. London: The Hogarth Press.

Freud, Sigmund. 1917. "Mourning and Melancholia." In *The Standard Edition of the Complete Psychological Works of Sigmund Freud*, edited and translated by James Strachey, vol. 14, 237–58. London: The Hogarth Press.

Freud, Sigmund. 1920. *Beyond the Pleasure Principle*. In *The Standard Edition of the Complete Psychological Works of Sigmund Freud*, edited and translated by James Strachey, vol. 18, 1–64. London: The Hogarth Press.

Gay, Peter. 1991. *Freud: A Life for Our Time*. London: Norton, 1988. Trans. into French by Tina Jolas as *Freud: Une Vie*, Paris: Hachette.

Laub, Dori. 1998. "The Empty Circle: Children of Survivors and the Limits of Reconstruction." *Journal of the American Psychoanalytic Association* 46 (2): 507–29.

Laub, Dori. 2005. "Traumatic Shutdown of Narrative and Symbolization: A Death Instinct Derivative?" *Contemporary Psychoanalysis* 41 (2): 307–26.

Laub, Dori, and Daniel Podell. 1995. "Art and Trauma." *International Journal of Psycho-Analysis* 76: 991–1005.

Papadopoulos, Renos. 2007. "Refugees, Trauma and Adversity-Activated Development." *European Journal of Psychotherapy and Counselling* 9 (3): 301–12.

Van der Kolk, Bessel. 2014. *The Body Keeps the Score: Brain, Mind, and Body in the Healing of Trauma*. New York: Viking.

Varvin, Sverre. 2019. "Psychoanalysis and the Situation of Refugees: A Human Rights Perspective." In *Psychoanalysis, Law and Society*, edited by Plinio Montagna and Adrienne Harris. Published by Routledge/CRC Press, May 21. Available online: https://www.crcpress.com/Psychoanalysis-Law-and-Society/Montagna-Harris/p/book/9780367194505.

8   Mourning and Nostalgia

The Question

I notice that refugees' thoughts and feelings about a possible desire and/
or obligation to return to their country are not touched upon – for example, if their asylum applications receive repeated negative responses. If this
question is not asked at all in the meeting with the therapist in circumstances where it would be expected to be asked, this avoidance allows the
compulsive repetition of the defense mechanisms of denial of reality and
dissociation.

For example, Amina received her second rejection of her asylum application while living without work for two years in a camp on the outskirts
of Athens, and was informed that a year ago her family was deported from
Turkey to their village in Syria. Amina was the only one who managed
to pass from Turkey to Lesvos, where she received her first rejection of
her asylum application. From Lesvos, she arrived, though without papers,
Athens. Her father died a few months ago, and she could not attend his
funeral.

In the session after the second rejection, Amina says she feels ashamed
to see women taking care of their children in the camp but does not say a
word about her absence from the lives of her children, her husband, and
her mother in the difficult times they are going through. She mostly talks
about the lives of others inside and outside the camp, complaining that she
is not allowed to get out of it and have her own money in Greece. Even if
there is a death sentence against her (which we do not know), if she returns
to her village, we would now expect her to be able to talk about feelings
of guilt toward her loved ones, feelings of nostalgia or sadness, and loneliness away from them. Why does the therapist ally himself in the defensive
denial of any relationship with Amina's objects without alluding to it? For
example, when Amina mentions her shame in scenes where women care
for their children, he could comment that these scenes seem familiar to her,
thus offering her the possibility of connecting with her past.

I also notice that when I raise the issue during supervision, therapists
and the caregivers' team, in general, are surprised (with some implicit
anger) as if it were taken for granted that we are allied with the part of the

DOI: 10.4324/9781003639022-9

refugee that makes enormous sacrifices and goes through superhuman trials to leave and stay away from their country of origin.

The question arises within me: Why we ally ourseives in the leaving entirely in the dark the always present conflict a refugee is confronted with at every turning point of his journey: to stay or to leave.His conscious decision has in general an internal, opposite side, an important one to talk about with a therapist.

On every relocation trip, there are issues of idealization and obsolescence, as well as splitting phenomena between the investment of the new host country and the old country from which someone has left. The influence of the new culture on the scale of values of the immigrant/refugee, the learning of a new language, and the interaction with people of different religions and politico-social beliefs are among the factors of transformation, not only of external behavior but also of the internal sense of the Self. The result can be attributed to a long period of hatching a new identity that, in the desired version, harmoniously combines old and newly acquired aspects, *a third individuation* according to the term proposed by Salman Akhtar (1995, 2016).

The above individuation presupposes the successful process of grieving for what someone has lost during the move. The mourning can be facilitated by a mostly welcoming reception of the immigrant from the country and society where he moved. Similarly, Kristin White, in *Migration and Integration in the Internal and External Community: Narcissistic Defense Organizations as a Hindrance to Integration* (2022), argues that for a migrant to feel that he belongs to the community of the country he is going to, he must have completed the mourning of all that he has left behind.

Like Salman Akhtar, Kristin White stresses that she is talking about migrants (those who have voluntarily left their respective countries). She considers that for some migrants with narcissistic defenses who do not easily turn to others to seek help and do not integrate into the host country's community, migration is a kind of mental refuge. The narcissistic defenses raised against the anxieties of the depressed position lead to a negative therapeutic response that creates difficulties and even discontinuation of treatment (Steiner 1993, 2020).

What about refugees whose reception is anything but welcoming? It is difficult for a migrant to mourn what he has left behind while preparing for his relocation, often for a long time, let alone for a refugee whose refugee route begins violently and unprepared and, often, without the possibility of return. Refugees who have been struggling for many years to survive without access to a private or often public mental health system do not have a treatment to interrupt for a long period of time.

In this chapter, starting from the case of Hekit, who decides to return to her country feeling for the first time the nostalgia for her homeland and the paternal family she left behind 17 years ago, I will focus on the phenomenon of nostalgia, the pain caused by the desire to return home.

Starting with the clinical material, I will ask whether a new identity is always created after an extended stay in the new country, or whether the mental shelter offered by migration functions as an enclave out of place and time.

Hekit's case is set at the crossroads of internal and external displacement. It shows how the internal displacement caused by the separation from her teenage daughter (during the daughter's second individuation) highlights the removal from primary, incestuous objects – one of the most painful tests of any individual development, contributing to the understanding of the extent of the painful experiences of each movement, including the refugee one.

Does caregivers' avoidance of focusing on the conflict between old and new identities take place on the defensive side of the sheer emotions that, in one way or another, may touch each one of us deep inside? Although it is not as devastating as the refugee route, it is still traumatic to another degree. Love for homeland has its first cores in childhood's primary emotions and performances. This is a record that none of the same is possible later. First impressions and first registrations will never be eliminated. The external world is inscribed in the inner world, which in turn transforms the outer one.

The therapist may be sure that he does not avoid the refugee's pain of longing to protect himself against his own nostalgia. Nostalgia can be felt as a danger for good reasons.

Nostalgia, after all, was seen as a disease, even potentially fatal, and not just as a common regime of a reactionary nature. Nostalgia has also been described as "impulsive insanity" in German ("Heimweh oder impulsives Irresein"; the word *Heimweh* appeared in the Swiss dialect in the seventeenth century). Although the words "nostalgo" and "nostalgia" sound absolutely Greek (from the word "nostos" and the word "algos," which means pain, suffering), they are not Greek. The word "nostalgia" is actually the name of a disease registered as such only in the seventeenth century. Johannes Hofer (1688) wrote a short medical dissertation on nostalgia as a disorder of the representational power that is constantly focused on the desire to return home so that no other psychic idea can be awakened. As associated with nostalgia, he considered the innermost part of the brain, which consists of countless nerve fibers. Nostalgia was expressed not only in the mental sphere but also in the body (Illbruck 2012).

Another version, according to the *Historical Dictionary of the French Language*, claims that Johann Jakob Harder (1656–1711), professor of medicine and botanist from Basel, coined the word nostalgia, in 1678, in order to name the pain of the homeland, *Heimweh*, from which the loyal, highly paid Swiss mercenaries of Louis 14th suffered; "The Swiss deserted the army when they heard bucolic melodies, this much-cherished tune of the Swiss," writes Rousseau in his Dictionary of Music, "hence it was forbidden under penalty of death to play these tunes in their ranks; because those who listened to it broke down into tears, deserted or died, so awakened in them the burning desire to see their homeland again" (Cassin, 2013, 29 and 30).

The etymology of the word *nostos* is not considered absolutely certain. The most authoritative etymological dictionaries trace it to the verb "neomai" (usually prepositioned with "from") from the same family as the verb "nesomai," of Indo-European root and meaning. The two related verbs mean the following: to arrive somewhere happily, to be saved from great danger or serious illness, to return, to return home. The noun "nostos" (and by extension the adjective "tasty," "nostimos" in Greek) converges the previous meanings, among which the last and final one stands out. Nostos therefore mainly means "return to the native land" (Maronitis et al. 2007).

Moreover, in the time of Karl Jaspers, the interest of the scientific community attracted certain crimes such as arson and murder that could be attributed to intense nostalgia, due to the incredible brutality and horrible determination with which they were committed. It was the above crimes that young Jaspers was interested in. His treatise *Nostalgia and Crime* was published in 1909, just two years before the completion of *General Psychopathology*. These were obviously borderline situations but, as is usually the case, the extreme occurrences described facilitate a fuller understanding of a disorder or mental response and thus promote the empathy necessary to understand milder mental states.

Going to a literary paradigm, *the Odyssey*, the epic of travel par excellence, there is a dominant choice from the start. Odysseus does not leave Ithaca but travels to return to it. At this point, it should be added that Athena, who urges Odysseus' son Telemachus at the beginning of the *Odyssey* to leave Ithaca in search of his father, pushes him to adopt the temporary abandonment of Ithaca as his father did. According to one version, Athena is the father himself. The father can help to correctly appreciate the archaic monsters of the journey – that is, the primary maternal images – by strengthening the fighting Ego against inner dangers. The beings of horror that can appear during the journey are comparable to the Sphinx faced by Oedipus. In both narratives, these are projections coming from the depths of prehistory and the unconscious. The therapist should join the refugee to face the crucial questions: Why he left, what he left behind, he still makes the choice of not returning if he has the possibility to do so. Through the following clinical material, I will try to show how, with the above avoidance, the therapist offers "kindness without truth" (Steiner 2020, 53ff). Even if this avoidance is needed as a period of preparation for the refugee to be able to face his truth later, the therapist should keep this goal in mind, not overlook it.

Clinical Material

The case of Hekit – and Dina: Dina is 18 years old, born in Greece to refugee parents from a North African country. Hekit was referred to the EPAPSY's team following a suicide attempt a few weeks after Dina graduated from school. At the meeting of the family with the psychologist, Dina mentioned that she had problems with her parents that confined her to home. In the meeting with the parents, the psychologist found out that the parents had come to Greece 20 years ago, as the family of Hekit did not accept this marriage.

The psychologist also realized that Dina was suffocating mainly under the supervision of her mother – the father seemed to be a calm, relatively passive man, especially tender with his elder daughter. Dina's mother, Hekit, is 50 years old and, relying on the traditions of Islam, expresses great objections to her daughter's "Western" lifestyle in Athens. The father is quite absent from home and cannot influence the relationship between the mother and the daughter. The mother seems too worried about the removal of the daughter from her. But the psychologist had exactly the opposite concern as she was informed by Dina that she still sleeps with her mother. At the same time, she found Dina –and her younger brother – smart, beautiful, talented, and sociable. The therapy team decided to offer the mother a series of 12 counseling psychotherapy sessions (with the possibility of more sessions if the therapist deems it necessary) so that she can allow her daughter to make the moves of independence and separation from an almost symbiotic relationship with her – moves of separation and individuation imposed on the late adolescent Dina from her biological and mental maturation. The team also decided to offer Dina a series of 12 counseling psychotherapy to help her toward constructing a plan for her studies and in general the entrance to her adult life.

The mother accepted, considering, in retrospect, that what she says to her own therapist will be transferred to her daughter's therapist, who will then act as her mouthpiece so that Dina will be pressured to remain "tied to" the mother. In fact, in her second session, Hekit boldly told her therapist: "tell Mrs. X this so she can tell my daughter." At the beginning of the session, Hekit expressed satisfaction with her daughter's progress by being calmer, not arguing with her. But she added that the psychologist should tell the daughter's therapist that she should be vigilant about a setback because her daughter is not trustworthy. Her therapist, annoyed by both Hekit's disbelief and authoritative tone, told her that she comes here for herself and that things cannot be done the way she imagines. She can tell her daughter something for Dina to tell her therapist, or she can ask for a direct meeting with Dina's therapist to tell her something, if the daughter agrees. To the surprise of the practitioner, who expected Hekit to get angry, hearing the above words, the mother seemed very moved. She cried asking: "So here I can talk about myself?" Receiving an affirmative answer from the therapist, she seemed very happy.

Hekit continued talking about her own body, her aging, and her hormonal tests. The practitioner was happy to think that a step had been taken toward investing herself and her body as separate from Dina, especially since Hekit seemed to be trying to speak for herself.

On supervision, however, I pointed out the anger the therapist expected from Hekit. Instead, a more mature and dispassionate reaction came, unexpected from what we knew about this mother and daughter's relationship. Nothing explained such a rapid improvement for a woman so attached to her daughter. It could only be a defensive flight to health.

In the session after that, Hekit spoke about her paternal family after asking: "So now I am *only* going to talk about myself?" Hekit spoke for the first time about her family in Morocco as if removing the possibility of having her daughter revealed her tenuous connection to Greece and the inadequacy of creating a new identity that includes elements of the new culture, although she has been living in Athens for 20 years. As she talked about her father back in Morocco, saying that they have good social and economic standing, she began to express strong nostalgia for her family back in the country where she had fled 20 years ago! Hekit added that with her father's help, she could get a good job with a few responsibilities to rebuild her life. Much to her surprise, the practitioner realized that Hekit was planning to return to her home country soon after she felt she had to separate from Dina. It would be inconceivable for her to stay in Greece with her husband and children if her daughter left the symbiotic relationship with her.

Hekit said her husband would never be able to find a job at this age in their country (sharing her father's underestimation of him and neglecting her son totally), adding that she is trying to convince Dina to follow her, where traditions keep her closer to her mother. Her great aggression and anger toward the therapist, who told her that she is separate from her daughter and can talk about herself, has now become apparent. There were cancellations of her subsequent sessions, and at the 12th and final session, where Hekit also canceled, the therapist contacted her to suggest they say goodbye to an additional session. Hekit accepted. She said goodbye by hugging her and told her that she was currently preparing to go back. Knowing that she will be bound entirely by traditions there, Dina does not want to follow her. That is why, she added, she saw no reason to come to the sessions. She prefers to think about what job she will do to make more money because she is too ashamed of herself at the point she has reached.

Hekit's psychologist was taken aback by the abrupt and unexpected interruption of her treatment "to return home." I found – in supervision – positive in this session that Hekit was able for the first time to compose the two places in her speech and say that many things hurt her in Morocco and that made her ashamed (the main one being that she did not have a marriage estimated by her family) but that in Greece she also experienced very significant losses. In other words, she could see the pros and cons of both countries. In the session after the psychologist's confrontation that she will not be her master's voice, that is, in the third session, she said to her therapist in a muffled voice: "So now I am going to talk only about myself?"

It was not enough for her to talk about herself in Greece if her daughter was not included in that self as a precious complement.

Hekit spoke of her siblings, who have a good social and economic standing, and announced her decision to return to a country she had never visited during her 20 years in Greece. Of course, she would leave her therapy and her husband and children. In a cold voice, she said that her husband would never be able to find a good job at that age in Morocco, while she, with the help of her father, could find a good job with few responsibilities and rebuild her life.

Regardless of whether or not she returned to Morocco, Hekit, through her daughter's mental process and the help of her psychologist, was able, for the first time, to face what she lost in Morocco and what coming to Greece meant and to start the work of mourning. The shame that she mentions accompanies the beginning of mourning and is a powerful and significant feeling for migrants and refugees. Hekit was able to acknowledge this with a therapist who perceived her in her human dimension, independent of her daughter, and insisted, despite the rejection of therapy, to say goodbye. A goodbye which she had not done until now in her old life.

Elements of Theory

Hekit's case is of particular interest because it shows, in a limited number of sessions, how the negative therapeutic response takes place not only interrupting the mother's counseling but also threatening the entire family edifice that was built up during 20 years in Greece. Hekit's anger is reminiscent of the myth of Demeter and Persephone, since she seems to blackmail the therapist by implicitly but clearly claiming that "since you cannot give me my daughter back, I will destroy everything, abandon you all and leave." In the above myth, the mother, mourning the loss of her daughter, who was kidnapped by Hades, blackmails Zeus, his brother and husband, by desolating the cultivation of the land and destroying agriculture. She asks him to intercede for the daughter to be returned to her. Did not Hekit expect the same from the therapists? To intercede and return her daughter to her bed and in her arms.

The treatment team did not clearly understand the depth and importance of the union of mother and daughter. The mother's therapist felt that a pedagogical approach would suffice to enlighten the mother that Dina's removal would benefit both of them. However, the mother could not follow her on this route. The status of the refugee route overlapped with Hekit's narcissistic difficulties that surfaced after the therapeutic team intervened to facilitate the kidnapping of Dina (Persephone) by Hekit (Demeter). The myth had the subterfuge of Persephone eating pomegranate seeds in the underworld that forced her to return for six months to her husband, abandoning her mother. The bond between mother and daughter was not eliminated but halved.

Apparently, prior to having Dina, there were intense incestuous ties for Hekit in her paternal family, and the presence of her husband was not able to sufficiently loosen them. He was powerful enough to take Hekit away from the country but only to give her the fruit she craved so much: children and especially, Dina, her beloved! If the children, and indeed the daughter, did not stay with her, he was someone who would not be able to stand by her. So, when Dina, with her graduation, initiated aid mechanisms to detach herself from her mother, Hekit had only to return to her homeland and in the arms of her paternal family.

Hekit's suicide attempt is reminiscent of Daren Aronofsky's film *Black Swan* (2010), where the daughter, in order to be removed from the nursery and the constant care and presence of the mother, self-harms, leaving the suspicion of a catastrophic triumph, an exit from the dual relationship of mother and daughter at the cost of her death. We can imagine that the graduation of Dina was for Hekit something like a catastrophic triumph toward her own mother left in Morocco (meaning her internal representation of her mother).

The pre-Oedipus bond between mother and daughter has attracted the interest of female psychoanalysts who complemented Freud's stance on the psychosexual development of women. Deutsch (1925), Horney (1924, 1926), and Lampl-de Groot (1927) were among the first to point out the importance of moving away from the dual relationship between mother and daughter to the triadic relationship involving the father of the Oedipal phase. Although the above issue is always timely and important – see, for example, Nancy Kulish and Deanna Holtzman's book *A Story of Her Own: The Female Oedipus Complex Reexamined and Renamed* (2008) – in this book we are intrigued because in my opinion, it highlights in retrospect how important it is to approach why someone leaves their home country, what he leaves behind, and what he seeks.

War, poverty, political persecution, and torture naturally overshadow anything else with their brutality and violence and often obscure the savagery and violence inherent in people's everyday situations. The need for the daughter to abandon the bond with the mother and "leave" toward the creation of her identity, toward the world of the father and objects other than the mother, is also a problematic refugee journey. If it is not done successfully enough, as in the case of Hekit, it will create an intergenerational transmission of the difficulty of separating. Dina was, for Hekit, a substitute for a previous relationship that presumably involved a member of her paternal family. Whatever Hekit lost by her daughter's removal made her feel ashamed. Now, she had to try to find a way to make money and find work to earn a substitute.

Another patient who visited me at my doctors' office visibly suffering from depression (as indicated by her drawn features and expressionless and icy face) said she wanted me to help her have sex with her husband. It was only when I asked for a relative to come with her next time that I was informed of what she could not tell me. Her daughter who accompanied her the second time had found a job abroad and would leave in the next few days. But this loss cannot easily be put into words and is cloaked in an interest in sex with the husband or in finding a job or protecting the daughter from the Western way of life.

To be able to accept a loss at present, we must confront the unresolved mourning of our past. If we have not completed the separations of our lives, the mental work of mourning each new loss will be hindered or even not at all (Volkan and Zintl 1993). Hekit, fleeing the pain of loss, turned back. She did not have enough strength to move forward, as she seemed to have hoped in the eighth session. She had unresolved issues, as seems to indicate the choice of daydreaming to return home. The more intense the nostalgia for reunion, the more violent the reaction to loss can be, as the crimes studied by Jaspers (1996 [1909]), Aronofsky's film, or the myth of Demeter and Persephone teach us. Illnesses, suicide attempts, pain, and recourse to alcohol or substances are among the potential risks that the therapist should keep in mind.

Bibliography

Akhtar, Salman. 1995. "A Third Individuation: Immigration, Identity and the Psychoanalytic Process." *Journal of the American Psychoanalytic Association* 43: 1051–1084.

Akhtar, Salman. 2016. Salman Akhtar on "A Third Individuation: Immigration, Identity and the Psychoanalytic Process." *PEP/UCL Top Authors Project Video Collection* 1: 17.

Cassin, Barbara. 2013. *La Nostalgie. Quand donc est-on chez soi? Ulysse, Énée, Arendt.* Paris: Éditions Autrement. Trans. into Greek by Cécile Inglessi Margelou as *Η Νοσταλγία: Πότε Είμαστε Στο Σπίτι Μας; Οδυσσέας, Αινείας, Άρεντ*. Athens: Ink Publications, 2015.

Deutsch, Helene. 1925. "The Psychology of Women in Relation to the Function of Reproduction." *International Journal of Psychoanalysis* 6: 405–18.

Hofer Johannes (1688). Dissertatio curioso-medicade Nostalgia-vulgo heimwehe oder heimsehnsucht, Th. IX , Basel.

Horney, Karen. (1924). "On the genesis of the castration complex in women." *International Journal of Psychoanalysis* 5: 50–65.

Horney, Karen. 1926. "The Flight from Womanhood." *International Journal of Psychoanalysis* 12: 360–374.

Illbruck, Helmut. 2012. *Nostalgia: Origins and Ends of an Unenlightened Disease.* Evanston, IL: Northwestern University Press.

Jaspers, Karl. (1996). *Heimweh und Verbrechen.* Munich: Belleville.

Kulish, Nancy, and Deanna Holtzman. 2008. *A Story of Her Own: The Female Oedipus Complex Reexamined and Renamed.* Lanham, MD: Jason Aronson.

Lampl-de Groot, Jeanne. 1927. "The Evolution of the Oedipus Complex in Women." *International Journal of Psychoanalysis* 9: 332–45.

Maronitis, Nikos D., and Lefteris Polkas. 2007. *Archaic Epic Poetry: From the Iliad to the Odyssey.* Athens: Triantafyllidis Foundation.

Silverman, Maxine. 2012. "On Myths and Myth-Making: Psychoanalytic Theorizing About Mother-Daughter Relationships and the "Female Oedipus Complex."" *Psychoanalytic Quarterly* 81 (3): 727–50.

Steiner, John. 1993. *Psychic Retreats. The New Library of Psychoanalysis*, vol. 19. London: Routledge.

Steiner, John. 2020. *Illusion, Disillusion, and Irony in Psychoanalysis*. London: Routledge.

Volkan, Vamik, and Elizabeth Zintl. 1993. *Life After Loss: The Lessons of Grief*. London: Routledge.

White, Kate. 2020. "Migration, Loss and Psychic Retreat." In *Migration and Intercultural Psychoanalysis*, edited by Kate White and Isabel Klingenberg, 30–43. London: Routledge.

White, Kate. 2022. "Migration and Integration in the Internal and External Community: Narcissistic Defense Organizations as a Hindrance to Integration." *International Journal of Psychoanalysis* 103 (1): 174–90.

Film

Black Swan. 2010. Directed by Darren Aronofsky. Written by Mark Heyman and Andres Heim. Los Angeles: Fox Searchlight Pictures.

9 Psychosis and Violence

The Question

Recurrent nightmares, sleep disturbance (difficulty falling or staying asleep), physical pain, self-injurious behavior, irritability, withdrawal and persistent difficulty in being involved in human relationships are common symptoms for refugees either in the first reception area or in their place of relocation. Each refugee develops a different pathology depending on his personality and, of course, depending on the degree of complexity of the new situation in which he finds himself. The loss of a secure network of relationships and, most importantly, the pressure from the need to adapt to an unfamiliar environment are stressors that contribute to the release of a mental illness.

In some refugees, mental illness may not appear immediately but years after settling in the new country. In other words, after a period of good adaptation, a period free of conflicts and symptoms, the psyche collapses either in the form of a psychotic break or in the form of a depressive or even borderline illness. In other refugees and/or migrants, mental illness occurs at the exact time of relocation.

For example, a 20-year-old Greek who went to a US university on a full scholarship because of his excellent mathematical thinking could not adapt to student groups. The jokes his farmer uncle told him sounded racist in Boston society and led to his isolation. Isolation caused the loss of a sense of self. The collapse of the self led to persecutory type's delusions with auditory and tactile hallucinations emanating from Chinese centers and channeling through electrical waves into his body – Chinese were many of his fellow students who rejected him from the football team on which the young student hoped to find a way to socialize.

The Grinbergs (Grinberg and Grinberg 1989, 145) consider that the onset of the disease after years may be contributed by the loss of the unconscious, deep belief that migration is transient. They cite the case of a 30-year-old woman who immigrated to the United States following her husband. Loneliness led her to the collapse of compulsive organization and corresponding defenses and paved the way for the emergence of a hallucinatory image where her son dissolved into pieces. During the pseudo-illusion

DOI: 10.4324/9781003639022-10

(she knows that it is a creation of her mind, so it is not a true illusion), the woman turned to the memory of her analyst to calm down, which is common in these situations, where someone is looking for an anchor to keep him from falling apart. "You needed to feel me close to feel whole," the seasoned analyst told her. Mental illness and, in the case that interests us in this chapter, a psychotic disorder may not be the result but the cause of constant migration.

In the case of Khalil that I will present, the constant flight from South Africa to Egypt, from there to Turkey and from Turkey to Lesvos and Athens was the result of a jealous type's delusional disorder that went undiagnosed, without medication and without any treatment and/or counseling to him and his wife on how to help him and be helped. How did Khalil's mental illness remain undiagnosed for so many years? The answer is that the refugee journey itself, the flight from place to place, was his subterfuge, his defensive reaction when he felt that he could not face the paranoid ideas that were created in the place where he lived and worked.

We have an amazing description of this defense by Robert Musil in The *Man Without Attributes,* the "psychoanalytic novel par excellence" as the psychoanalyst Johannes Cremerius called it. Musil writes:

As long as he (the hero) kept others at a distance, as was always the case in the beginning, with his laconic, friendly calm and intense industriousness, he stayed; as soon as they began to treat him with intimacy and without respect, as if they had already known him, he left, because then a terrible feeling overwhelmed him, as if he did not feel confident in his skin. ... Once he was late in doing so; then four builders in a building conspired to make him feel their superiority by throwing him down the upper floor of the scaffolding; he heard them giggling behind his back and approaching, and then he threw himself with all his unlimited strength upon them, threw one or two staircases down, and cut the tendons of the arm of two others. The punishment for his act shook his soul, as he said. He emigrated to Turkey, and then back again, because the whole world had rallied against him; no magic refrain could fight this conspiracy, and no kindness.

(pp. 84–85)

The narcissistic fragility of Musil's hero is excellently described in the above quote, highlighting *the principle of the hammock,* that is, the need to choose the right distance between the psychotic subject and others, therefore the therapist as well.

Psychoanalytic theory holds that the loss of boundaries between the Ego and the Object leads to the collapse of the Ego due to the fusion with the Object, so in order to protect himself, the psychotic patient moves away from the Object. But then the ego disappears again because of complete withdrawal from the Object. Between these two positions as to the Object, the psychotic walks *on a narrow strip of land*, as this is graphically depicted in an image. In this strip of land, the patient struggles to survive mentally – and often physically – through a constant battle with psychotic illness (Giannoulaki 2021). In other words, the psychotic patient is confronted with the fundamental contradiction between self-oriented and object-oriented tendencies (Mentzos 2002, 103). It is not a conflict as we know them from neuroses, but another type of conflict, and the patient's delirium is a kind of compromise. It is not only a projection of intrapsychic aggression, but also the maintaining of a kind of relationship between persecutor and persecuted, a kind of compromise between wanting contact with the object and defending against it. For example, Khalil mauled the interpreter during the first visit of the team to their apartment.

The therapist spoke during supervision about Khalil and asked for help because he frightened her with his loss of control over his behavior and the confusion leading to difficulty to understand his pathology. The therapist, who was proven to have a great capacity for empathy for her patients, was particularly angry at Khalil's violent behavior toward his wife; she felt that she was dealing with yet another behavior of violence toward women that can end in femicide, a male behavior so common among refugees coming from South Africa. Violence toward women and the risk of femicide was not an accidental association of the therapist. However, at the same time, it does not belong to Khalil's present situation but to another relative and femicide in his biography, as will be shown by the clinical material.

His silent acceptance of his wife did not help to estimate his beliefs' bizarre or unnatural nature. Lynne Layton (2006) refers to "normative unconscious processes" that characterize "those aspects of the unconscious that are the psychological consequence of living in a cultural environment in which many norms serve the dominant ideological goal of maintaining the status quo." The case of Rosa and her son from Eisold (Eisold 2019, 94–6), where Rosa wonders if she should allow her son to abuse her like his father, to help him "be a man," highlights the fear that if the man is not abusive toward the woman, he is himself a "woman" sheds lights on this issue.

In this case also, there is a need for a diagnosis. Is Khalil's belief of his wife betraying him a symptom of psychosis?

Khalil's case highlights the possible relationship between trauma and psychosis by overturning the thesis that psychosis is inaccessible by the psychodynamic approach and the pessimism it generates in new therapists when confronted with it (Knafo and Selzer 2024).

In one sentence, the question of this chapter is the following: If (refugee) caregivers' desire to heal refugees is strengthened by their identification with their suffering fellow man, how can they be helped if the beneficiary of their care subject presents a psychotic pathology, and hence, they find it challenging to recognize similarities between them and the patient? Moreover, if there is so often the need to differentiate a symptom as being a psychotic one or not, a good enough knowledge of the psychosis is not desirable for the refugees' caregivers?

There is no doubt, however, that, especially for the psychotic refugee, the supervision of caregivers is necessary because in order to ensure the best possible treatment for the refugee, it is a prerequisite to help the caregiver endure the difficult emotions that the combination of psychosis and trauma causes.

Clinical Material

The social services of the camp asked for Khalil's evaluation and treatment after a suicide attempt following an intense argument with his wife. Khalil seems confused, disorganized, and his speech is slightly incoherent. He surprises the therapist because he does not refer to a feeling of depression or hopelessness but instead says with an inappropriate affect that he "saw" his wife dating with a neighbor. At that moment, he thought that the doctor was not able to help him.

The practitioner lost it hearing this. So, was he taking psychiatric drugs? She asked him, and he replied surprised and annoyed that, of course, he is on antidepressant medication. He needed the drugs to be able to satisfy his wife sexually; otherwise, she is looking for a lover. Therefore, it is better for him to die than to be shamed by the unfaithful woman. He said to the psychologist that he wished he did not know any of this. He wished his wife did it secretly!

The psychologist was horrified by his account and asked for him to be referred to the team's psychiatrist who diagnosed paranoid psychotic disorder. His wife, he told the psychiatrist, often yelled at him, when they argued, that he was crazy. Calling the woman to give his history, the psychiatrist realized that his wife, as is often the case, did not mean that he is crazy in the psychiatric sense of the disease, but in the characterological trait of a jealous husband who goes mad with jealousy – something that because it was in line with the usual possessive attitude of men in South Africa did not attract any special attention from her. For the denial of violence and madness I will talk more extensively in the part on the theory of this chapter. It quickly became apparent that Khalil never received proper treatment, since his illness was never diagnosed by a psychiatrist. Instead, Khalil resorted to a journey from country to country to deal with his illness, moving away from any place where he perceived his wife flirting with a man.

It began in South Africa, where Khalil saw his wife flirting with his brother. Then, in Egypt, where the family arrived to move away from this brother and meet another relative, Khalil started the same thing again and asked his relative to swear in the Qur'an that he sees his wife as a sister and not romantically. His relative replied that he was crazy, but, as the account shows, there was never any question of taking him to a psychiatrist. They got into a violent fight, and Khalil fled to Turkey with his wife and children for fear of killing his relative. At the border, Turkish border guards arrested them and deported them back to South Africa, where they lived for the next two years. Khalil then "found out" that his wife was cheating on him with one of her cousins, and since his relative had left for Germany, they returned to Egypt. Three years later, he "realized" that his wife was having an affair with the owner of the apartment where they lived and set off again for Turkey. They then decided to come to Greece on their way to Germany, where other relatives already live.

The psychologist who treated Khalil told the supervision team that during their meetings, she felt terrible physically. Khalil's constant change of subject and intensity caught her up in something of vertigo. She felt he was dangerous. His danger was confirmed when, between sessions offered by the psychologist, Khalil was put in jail for badly beating the social worker of the facility. The social service decided to pay bail to get Khalil out of jail.

With the help of supervision, supporting the stance that even in such a serious disease, the offer of a therapeutic relationship focused on treating the refugee patient as a human subject whose biography matters and is explored with empathy and respect, the therapeutic team decided to offer Khalil a series of psychotherapeutic sessions.

During therapy, Khalil told the psychologist that he spoke to someone about his life for the first time. He was relieved and grateful that someone listened to his story without judging.

Khalil said that they moved to South Africa from Iran. They were Muslims, a minority in South Africa. His father died when he was 5 and his mother was married with a local after some years. It all started with the murder of his mother by his stepfather, in front of his eyes, when he was 10. The stepfather entered with a long outfit, inside which he hid the gun, and shot her several times. His stepfather was old and sick. His mother was young and beautiful and had lovers in the city. Khalil, her youngest son and most beloved, wished for years that his mother would not take him with her, a witness to her love life! Khalil remembers seeing her lovers hold her in their arms and being jealous. He remembers his mother being late, leaving him waiting, and feeling anxious while she was with her lovers. He also remembers that after his father's death, Khalil asked her if she married another, and they all stayed together. She promised him and seemed happy.

But the stepfather had other plans and killed her to wash away the shame. He was forced to pretend to agree with the murder or he would be an outcast in society. He would not be a man and would be in danger of being abused in numerous ways by the men of the small society where he lived, having lost for good both the protection and affection of his mother.

Khalil sighs and tells the therapist that he wishes she knew none of this, reminding her of the wish he had expressed at their first meeting that she knew nothing of his wife's infidelities. Khalil said that he leaves every time he fears that he will become like his stepfather and kill the unfaithful woman!

The symmetry of delirium and trauma became evident, and the therapist strengthened her capacity for empathy and understanding. She felt she offered Khalil a human relationship that could potentially be a stepping stone out of the lonely world he had entered after his mother's murder. The futility and helplessness that the therapist had felt at first subsided, enhancing the curiosity of the group members for our psychotic fellow human beings.

Elements of Theory

Khalil "sees" his wife dating a neighbor, "hears" being told that they are having an affair. Is this an illusion?

The point is that we must know the biography and the culture from which the refugee come to be able to decide if there is a psychotic disorder or not. In the article *Mourning and Issues of Identity in the Treatment of Refugees in Lesvos* (Christopoulos et al. 2021), we presented the case of Mr A, a 25-year-old man from Congo hearing voices and seeing ghosts. We found out that the hallucinatory symptoms had meaning that needed to be clarified. The knowledge of complicated mourning, or the *Ulysses syndrome*, noted in the literature (Achotegui 2019; Akhtar 1999), particularly with respect to guilt, enabled the understanding of the meaning of the ghosts (Christopoulos et al. 2021, 128).

A similar case where the hearing of voices was not a psychotic symptom is presented by Barbara Eisold. In the case of Ms. A, "the voice of Allah in her head gave her a sense of power, the sort of power 'fathers' in her culture might have assumed" (Eisold 2019, 85).

Nonetheless, even, after deciding that the refugee suffers from a psychotic symptom, caregivers still have to explore the symptom and find ways to work with the above patient who is in extreme emotional distress (Ophir 2015).

This chapter's patient, Khalil, perceives with certainty something that does not exist, in other words perceptual data is created without there being an external, sensory, stimulus. However, after the biographical data that Khalil offered in his treatment, we can think that in his delirium is expressed his vital mental side which he had not been able to integrate, which was dissociated, concerning the femicide of his mother by her second husband after the death of Khalil's father. Therefore, he ended up "living" it through his psychosis, searching for his own power "father" who can satisfy his wife instead of him who feels powerless.

It is a well-known theoretical thesis that in psychosis the history and continuity of the patient's life are broken. But in Khalil the emergence of the biographical element in symptomatology is evident.

Khalil lives at this exact area of his life in a reality of his own, and no argument or proof from his wife or anyone else can convince him of the baselessness of his own conception of reality, because there is a kernel of truth in his delirium, but it concerns another woman in another time that haunts his present. We know that in the case of a traumatic situation the senses form a timeless, motionless, mythically shaped traumatic background that can return at each moment, as always present.

The case of Khalil confirms the psychodynamic position that treats delirium as the conclusion of a secret psychic history:

> The psychotherapeutic approach to delirium generally consists in treating it as a symbol, in recognizing it as the conclusion of a secret psychic history. We must recognize that delirium is an act of self-affirmation of the patient resulting from his search for identity.
>
> (Benedetti 2002, 26)

Memory and truth, fantasy in its conscious and unconscious forms, and the relationship between mnemonic traces and constructions occupied Freud from the beginning to the end of his work (Masson 1985; Freud 1937). According to the Freudian view, not everyone or not always one has the ability to narrate their past, some "experience" it in the Here and Now. For example, Freud writes to Fliess, in the letter dated January 24,1897: "There is a class of people who to this very day tell stories like those of the withches and of my patients; hey are not believed, although their faith in their stories is not ot be shaken. As you have guessed, I mean paranoiacs, whose complaints that excrement is put in their food, that they are maltreated at night in the most shameful way sexually, an so on, are pure memory content." Freud returns to nonpsychotic illusions and connects them to memory in his 1937 article on Constructions, where he reasserts that there is a historical truth that is at the core of delirium, both individual and collective.

There are many psychodynamic models that attempt to understand psychosis within the Freudian tradition but also many psychological theories beyond it, starting with E. Bleuler, who (together with C. Jung and others) investigated in which psychotics it is possible to understand the significance of their symptoms in order to pave the way to discussion with them, and therefore toward psychotherapy.

The therapist's first goal is to develop and maintain the Therapeutic Alliance. Frank and Gunderson (1990), in the Boston Psychotherapeutic Study, examined the role of the therapeutic alliance in the course and outcome of 143 patients with schizophrenia and found that the therapeutic alliance was the decisive predictor of therapeutic success.

It is neither easy nor understandable for the therapist to acknowledge what the psychotic patient needs in order to feel secure in the relationship with the therapist. Various techniques have been formulated that aim to enhance the therapist's ingenuity in offering his psychotic patient himself as an object that is as little threatening as possible. In other words, knowledge of techniques is needed to help the therapist become sensitive to the perception of what causes terror to the psychotic in the relationship, forcing him to withdraw. I have already presented the importance of adjusting the distance: neither too close, nor too far.

The patient's own effort to deal with the disease (here the constant flight, and of course the delirium) is recommended to be treated with respect. Through the understanding of schizophrenic symptoms as attempts to combat the disease, the desire of the therapist to cooperate with the healthy parts of the ego of the schizophrenic that survive even the heaviest crises is reinforced. The cooperation of the therapist with the healthy part of the personality of the schizophrenic will prepare the ground for the future processing of the crisis at a later time and will strengthen the patient's self-healing powers.

Frese (1997), a successful psychologist who himself suffered from schizophrenia for many years, advised clinicians to avoid questioning patients' delusional beliefs. The avoidance of questioning delirium, although supported by public opinion (we do not say "no" to the madman), is not easily achieved because the therapist has to balance between maintaining an attitude of respect for delirium but at the same time a diligent avoidance of cooperation with the affected part of the patient.

In psychotic disorders, the concept of tact is particularly important. For example, the therapist should point out the pathological nature of an idea or behavior, without manifesting a position himself, to allow the patient to feel safe with him, even if he disagrees with the position the therapist puts in the mouth of others. He may, for example, make his observation as follows: *Therapist:* Some would say that you speak with a lot of love and admiration for your mother while being so angry that she subjected you to meetings that put you in a dangerous position.

The defense mechanism of denial is often found both in psychosis and in violence in general – not only in the victims of violence but also in all those involved. The tolerance and inadequate acknowledgment of violence is strongly observed in the female victim, as here in Khalil's wife. The above phenomenon is a puzzling fact, recognized especially in the field of violence against women.

Many psychoanalysts who have dealt with psychosis have emphasized the development of defenses against the psychotic experience that develops in therapy. There are several theories to explain the type and source of the therapist's defenses against his psychotic patient. Generally, the constant effort to understand the patient and his symptoms, even for defensive reasons, can prove to be a good tool under certain conditions: for example, if the therapist keeps in mind that his "cognitive projections" are a way to build bridges between the patient and him, to create a product of exchange, to start a "chat" that establishes a "transitional subject" (Benedetti 1998).

The subject of psychosis is too vast to explore in depth here, but we can introduce the caregivers to how they can work when encountering a refugee experiencing psychosis.

Selzer and Carsky (1990) emphasize the importance for a psychotic of finding an object that organizes, whether it is a person, an idea, or an inanimate object. For them, the advent of a therapeutic effect presupposes the active participation of the therapist, because the latter functions as a representative of a higher level of organization and is its mediator to the analysand.

More generally, psychodynamically oriented clinical work with psychotic patients supports the view that although in psychosis, and especially in schizophrenia, there are often early interpersonal difficulties (especially in the child–parent relationship), the ability to establish interpersonal relationships is preserved even in the most withdrawn patient (Sullivan 1962).

Although the above direction in the encounter with the schizophrenic allows us to get rid of the indifference to the human subject that we have in front of us – indifference that partly comes from the lack of investment he shows toward us – it is not enough for someone to carry out his therapeutic work, because in the case of schizophrenia, knowledge is required for this complex disease and experience in communicating with the schizophrenic and tools of psychodynamic direction. The therapeutic alliance can be achieved through the therapist's willingness in *"being with"* (McGlashan and Keats 1989) the schizophrenic, respecting his defenses, accepting thoughts of the schizophrenic even though he does not understand them, as well as his feelings, not attempting to change him possessed by excessive therapeutic claims.

It is important that the therapist seeks his own defenses that are mobilized in the encounter with the psychotic patient. It does not cease to be a fact, however, that the shared reality causes discomfort for all of us (as Freud highlighted in *Civilization and Its Discontents*) which, due to his disorder, the psychotic patient stirs within us, resulting in the mobilization of our defenses. An important defense consists in resorting to therapeutic action instead of connecting with the most personal data of the patient, his biography, psychotic symptoms, his experience.

In conclusion: Although it is an undeniable fact that psychoanalytic theory of psychoses does not occupy a central place today, it is an equally undeniable fact that it can contribute significantly for the clinician to be prepared for the abrupt entry of psychosis in the treatment room or the refugees' clinical – and it often does. The prepared therapist is familiar with the peculiarities of the psychotic patient and the particular techniques required.

Finally, I would like to add that in the supervision group, art helped, and we looked back on it to get hope and courage. This is achieved because art creates a global communication structure and helps significantly in cases where caregivers come from many different educational backgrounds,

bearing insufficiently metabolized theoretical positions that hinder communication. For example, in cinema, the film *A Beautiful Mind*, which
describes the life of the mathematician John Nash, who won the Nobel
Prize for his work in economics in 1994, reminds us understandably and
realistically that very important people can suffer from psychosis but, if
they are lucky and have the appropriate support, they will be able to cope
quite well with their lives.

Accepting, of course, the limits of human understanding of phenomena
as complex and primary as psychosis, I think it is good to remember that
even in such difficult mental conditions, psychoanalysis has broadened people's perception in the context of human encounters and communication.

Bibliography

Achotegui, Joseba. 2019. "Migrants Living in Very Hard Situations: Extreme
Migratory Mourning (the Ulysses Syndrome)." *Psychoanalytic Dialogues* 29 (3):
252–68.

Akhtar, Salman. 1999. "The Immigrant, the Exile, and the Experience of Nostalgia."
Journal of Applied Psychoanalytic Studies 1 (2): 123–30. https://doi.org/10.1023/A
:1023029020496.

Bachmann, Stefan, Franz Resch, and Christoph Mundt. 2003. "Psychological
Treatments for Psychosis." *Journal of the American Academy of Psychoanalysis* 31:
155–76.

Benedetti, Gaetano. 1998. *Le Sujet Emprunté: Le Vécu Psychotique du Patient et du
Thérapeute*. Paris: Éditions Érès, Coll. La Maison Jaune.

Benedetti, Gaetano. 2002. *La Psychothérapie des Psychoses Comme Défi Existentiel*.
Paris: Éditions Érès, Coll. La Maison Jaune.

Bleuler, Eugen. 1950. *Dementia Praecox or the Group of Schizophrenias*. 1911. Reprint,
New York: International Universities Press.

Christopoulos, Anna, Giannoulaki, Chrysi, Tzavaras, Nikolaos. 2021. "Mourning
and Issues of Identity in the Treatment of Refugees in Lesvos." In *Trauma, Flight,
and Migration: Psychoanalytic Perspectives*, edited by IPA in the Community.
London and New York: Routledge.

Dupont, Judith. 1988. "Ferenczi's 'Madness.'" *Contemporary Psychoanalysis* 24:
250–261.

Eisold, Barry K. 2019. *Psychodynamic Perspectives on Asylum Seekers and the Asylum-
Seeking Process: Encountering Well-Founded Fear*. London and New York:
Routledge.

Frank, Andrew F., and John G. Gunderson. 1990. "The Role of the Therapeutic
Alliance in the Treatment of Schizophrenia: Relationship to Course and
Outcome." *Archives of General Psychiatry* 47: 228–36.

Frese, Frederick J. 2000. "Recovery: Myths, Mountains, and Miracles." Presentation
to Menninger Clinic Staff, May 30, 1997. In *Psychodynamic Psychiatry in Clinical
Practice*, edited by Glen O. Gabbard. Washington and London: American
Psychiatric Publishing.

Freud, Sigmund. 1911. "The Case of Schreber." In *The Standard Edition of the Complete
Psychological Works of Sigmund Freud*, edited and translated by James Strachey,
vol. 12, 3–85. London: The Hogarth Press.

Freud, Sigmund. 1914. "On Narcissism: An Introduction." In *The Standard Edition of
the Complete Psychological Works of Sigmund Freud*, edited and translated by James
Strachey, vol. 14, 73–102. London: The Hogarth Press.

Freud, S. (1937). Constructions in Analysis. S.E. *Internationale Zeitschrift fur Psychoanalyse* 23 (4): 459–470.

Freud, Sigmund. 2002. "Studies on Hysteria." In *The Standard Edition of the Complete Psychological Works of Sigmund Freud*, vol. 2, 1895. Translated into Greek by L. Anagnostou as *Μελέτες για την Υστερία*. Athens: Epicurus Publications.

Gabbard, Glen O. 2000. *Psychodynamic Psychiatry in Clinical Practice*. Washington, London: American Psychiatric Publishing. Translated into Greek by Thomas Yfantis. Athens: Beta Publications.

Giannoulaki, Chrysi. 2021. "Schizophrenia Spectrum and Other Psychotic Disorders." In *Textbook of Psychodynamic Psychiatry*, edited by Stelios Stylianidis. Athens: Topos Books.

Grinberg, León, and Rebeca Grinberg. 1989. *Psychoanalytic Perspectives on Migration and Exile*. New Haven and London: Yale University Press.

Hartokollis, Peter. 1986. *Introduction to Psychiatry*. Athens: Foundation Publications.

Hinshelwood, R. D. 2004. *Suffering Insanity*. East Sussex: Brunner-Routledge.

Karon, Bertram P. 1992. "The Fear of Understanding Schizophrenia." *Psychoanalytic Psychology* 9: 191–211.

Keith, Stuart J., and Susan M. Matthews. 1984. "Schizophrenia: A Review of Psychosocial Treatment Strategies." In *Psychotherapy Research: Where Are We and Where We Should Go?*, edited by John B. W. Williams and Robert L. Spitzer. New York: Guilford.

Knafo, Danielle, and Marc Selzer. 2024. *From Breakdown to Breakthrough: Psychoanalytic Treatment of Psychosis*. New York: Routledge.

Layton, Lynne. 2006. "Racial Identities, Racial Enactments, and Normative Unconscious Processes." *Psychoanalytic Quarterly* 75: 237–69.

Masson, J. M. (1985). The complete letters of Sigmund Freud to Wilhelm Fliess, 1887-1904. Harvard University Press: London.

McGlashan, Thomas H., and Calvin J. Keats. 1989. *Schizophrenia: Treatment Process and Outcome*. Washington, DC: American Psychiatric Press.

Mentzos, Stavros. 2002. "I Disturbi Nevrotici Come Elaborazione Patologica del Conflitto." *Psicoterapia e Scienze Umane* 36 (1): 45–58.

Musil, R. 1987. *Der Mahn ohne Eigenschaften (1930, 1933, 1943). The man without Qualities*. Translated by Sieti, Toula. Vol. I. Athens: Odysseus publications.

Ophir, O. (2015). *Psychosis, psychoanalysis and psychiatry in postwar USA: On the borderland of madness*. Routledge.

Reich, Wilhelm. 1927. "A Hysterical Psychosis in Statu Nascendi." *International Journal of Psychoanalysis* 8: 159–73.

Searles, Harold F. 1965. "The Effort to Drive the Other Person Crazy—An Element in the Etiology and Psychotherapy of Schizophrenia." In *Collected Papers on Schizophrenia and Related Subjects*. 1959. Reprint, New York: International Universities Press.

Selzer, Marc A., and Carsky, Marc. 1990. "Treatment Alliance and the Chronic Schizophrenic." *American Journal of Psychotherapy* 44: 506–15.

Sullivan, Harry Stack. 1962. *Schizophrenia as a Human Process*. New York: Norton.

Film:

A Beautiful Mind. 2001. Directed by Ron Howard. Writers: Akiva Goldsman and Sylvia Nasar. Universal Pictures.

10 Ruptures and Reconstructions

The Question

In this chapter, the third and last one on caregivers' group supervision, I will try to address the tension between the individual refugee's right to be understood and the society's need or obligation to provide programs to host and help them – or to push them back – as a tension between understanding and explaining, metaphorically speaking.

In Chapter 1, I quoted Devereux as arguing that there is a complementary series' relationship between sociological explanation (involving an external observer) and psychological interpretation (involving an internal observer) (Devereux 2015). In the sciences of nature, man explains. In the interpretative tradition, man understands. Psychoanalysis has highlighted the separation of the concept of explanation from the concept of understanding, prioritizing the latter over the former.

Throughout this book, I insist on the need to understand, which often is obscured by the need to explain. Speaking about adult-onset trauma, Boulanger states from the same point of view:

> Rigorous attention to the patient's experience must take precedence over any preexisting theory of mind. Invoking early conflict, developmental arrests, or childhood trauma as an explanation for the alienation of adult-onset trauma is tantamount to blaming the victim, which is a political position. It should not be psychoanalytic.
>
> (Boulanger 2007, 180)

My active involvement with refugees began when the MDM caregivers' team expanded to meet the needs in Moria so much that a cohesive force was needed to absorb the vibrations created both by the arrival of the massive wave of refugees and by the abrupt and continuous changes in the number and organization of workers (Giannoulaki 2023).

The European refugee crisis has constituted the most significant wave of migration since World War II (Doctors of the World 2021a). According to the May 2021 UNHCR report, 89,000 people received international protection

DOI: 10.4324/9781003639022-11

in Greece between January 2016 and April 2021. The main entrance point was the island of Lesvos-Mytilene (Doctors of the World 2021b).

In cases where a large number of refugees leads to the need to "solve the refugees' problem," "strategies" and "systems" for managing mass influxes of people are constructed at a global level (Marrus 1985), ending in a contemporary narrative that fails to look at people as actual subjects: people with hopes, needs, and individual identities (Papadopoulos 2019, 32).

My hiring as a supervisor for the group of MDM carers was based on restoring the center of gravity to the individual and his particular personality and biography. As utopian as it may seem, the special interest of psychoanalytic theory and research in each individual – whether this person is a refugee, a camp worker, or a resident of the reception area – is a prerequisite for satisfactory work in the refugee field.

On the one hand, the funding for caring for the refugees, the immigration laws, and the process of evaluation of the asylum applications have their source in the fabric of society. So, some prioritize action, political or other. Seeley, for example, insists that a government that places responsibility for treating traumatic sequelae in clinics and individual consulting rooms evades the final responsibility for having created the conditions under which violence occurs in the first place (Seeley 2005). This explanation is based on the observation of objective reality.

On the other hand, as a psychoanalyst, I am concerned with the individual trying to listen not only to the unconscious, meaning to what is dissociated and split off, but also to what is still unrepresented and unable to be thought. This is the understanding through the psychoanalyst's conscious, preconscious, and unconscious experience during the initial individual consultation and later individual and group psychotherapies (Christopoulou et al. 2023).

Working with refugees and their carers does not allow for avoiding the tension between understanding and explaining between the individual and the general, which sometimes risks conflict. Paraphrasing Boulanger, I would say that we cannot and should not work from the position of the general, but in the case of the refugees, there is often pressure to do so (Boulanger 2007, 170). During my decade of working in the refugee field, I have often been confronted with turbulence within an NGO's caregivers' team, between NGOs, NGOs, and the political and social programs, or between the government and the community where they receive and care for refugees. I have already presented myself becoming "cruel" toward the team of carers in a facility for teenagers unaccompanied minors. Moreover, I sometimes felt anger, feeling that I, myself, am treated like a Xenos: someone whom they think is dangerous and immoral – for example, when some people did not allow me to refer to our collaboration in the refugee field.

Empathy is the tool for collecting psychoanalytic knowledge in the usual context of psychoanalysis. In the refugees' case, it becomes a sine qua non principle of caring for people who have experienced the unthinkable;

hence, their experiences remain unspeakable, unthought, unknown, and unrepresented. Marianne Leuzinger-Bohleber in the video (2021)1(1):35 "What Can Psychoanalysis Contribute to the Current Refugee Crisis" (IJP 2016) elevates empathy to the second principle on which he relied for the creation of Michaelis-Dorf Village. The first is security. On empathy, Dr Leuzinger-Bohleber said that it was crucial, as we already know from the camps of the displaced persons, what followed when they came out of the concentration camps. "They had an atmosphere of latent sadism again. Then they broke down, and we had many suicides. They lost the rest of hope. That was the second principle, to have empathy for the individual fate of this" (Leuzinger-Bohleber 2021).

However, can you just ask workers to empathize with refugees? Rather than encouraging understanding of the experience, sometimes crises that invite the public gaze and political attempts to "solve the problem" create situations where people cease to be subjects, becoming objects of curiosity or statistics instead. How can you enhance the ability of people– here, the caregivers – to be empathetic toward others – here, the refugees?

I believe that man understands constantly, even if he does not want to. Even if he does not attempt it intentionally, man cannot but form an opinion about the world around him (and therefore about his interlocutor) and himself as part of this world. In addition, though, man can deny or disavow what he understands. The above defense is one of the strongest in man when faced with trauma, therefore with something that overflows by definition, his psyche. In the above-mentioned video, Leuzinger-Bohleber characterizes the mechanism as a biologically rooted mechanism that pushes even those with the best intentions to "make techniques to put the people out of that. They make techniques to put the people into distance, they do not have to listen to them carefully, and to hear about what they have gone through" (Leuzinger-Bohleber 2021). When the above techniques that Leuzinger-Bohleber talks about are taught, the theory created within the subject who receives the above perspective can push you toward abandoning the spontaneous movement of the psyche toward the other.

Psychodynamically oriented supervision aims to facilitate movement toward the other, initially turning toward introspection, the understanding of our own experience. For the above reason, in critical moments, moments of rupture, even in the supervision team where we dealt each time with a particular refugee, we left all the time to detect and freely express as much as possible the feelings, fantasies, and thoughts of each of us.

No thought and speech can exist without considering man's emotional reaction that precedes it. Both categories of emotion and thought are indispensable tools in any attempt to analyze reality. Although man's movement toward the other is self-evident and spontaneous, humans need to learn to turn to what they feel inside them, which will inform them about what is happening to their fellow man whom they have undertaken to take care of.

Refugees, from the psychiatrist to the gatekeeper, are cared for by people, and the human dimension should not be ignored. By the way, I was delighted when the guard at the Moria gate approached me, asking if he could talk to me, too. Unfortunately, I could not respond, but if I had a group of psychodynamically minded graduate students, we might have been able to respond.

To sum up the problem:

On the one hand, refugee care facilities do not face a stable phenomenon over time, and they do not wish to hire employees who consider their work with refugees a permanent job, with all the consequences that this may have.

On the other hand, there can be no empathy from people who experience an unfair and inhumane attitude toward themselves. For example, especially when the waves of refugees are large, working conditions are exhausting for caregivers.

Also, more involvement is needed with residents, who often feel that refugees are better cared for than they are.

Last but not least, the media itself undermines the efforts of caregivers or the residents' reactions. Refugees, carers, and residents find themselves often represented in the media or hear about them in a way that destabilizes them. "Horror has a pornography of its own," states Boulanger (Boulanger 2007, 170). She adds: "The need for mastery compels fascination; terror at the ultimate futility of pitting oneself against contingency fuels repulsion" (ibid).

Therefore, allowing employees to express their anger, despair, and aggression and be contained is a unique way to counter the above.

I would like to add that the possibility of an empathetic attitude toward seriously injured people is not self-evidently available to everyone, and the above availability needs to be explored by anyone who wants to work in the refugee field.

I will take as a starting point the clinical material from these moments of rupture in supervision with a team of caregivers.

Clinical Material

During the supervision of a team of therapists, there were times when they asked or suggested that we do not deal with a refugee but with the group's feelings. The first time was when the head of the group had to choose one of the psychologists to be dismissed because of economic restrictions. He chose the oldest psychologist in the group because she could support herself professionally more quickly than the younger ones. Although the psychologist felt sad and had to say goodbye to the refugees she had in treatment within a month, we were able to make a touching farewell where we had the mental space to deal with the referral of her patients to someone else. The above psychologist was able to progress professionally.

In the above case, the coordinator participated in the supervision group – something I found particularly useful, as he knew the feelings of the caregivers from the individual supervision he gave to each member of the group, where he had the opportunity to deal with each caregiver individually. The above possibility was given by the small number of caregivers and by the stability of the program that had been taking place in Athens for some years.

On Lesvos, on the other hand, I was faced with unexpected redundancies that upset the team and created great insecurity. I recall the first operating principle that Leuzinger-Bohleber stood for, which was safety. For example, an interpreter was unexpectedly dismissed when he had just rented an apartment to stay on the island and work in Moria.

I think that the violence of uprooting refugees contributes to the fact that those working with refugees are themselves at risk of becoming violent in one way or another. The interpreter must have been prepared not to rent space while he is about to be made redundant.

Of course, neither an NGO nor a government can respond to the needs and problems of refugees. It seems inevitable to hurt either a refugee, a caregiver, or a neighbor. However, despair and guilt, when shared, become less traumatic and can be experienced as an inevitable part of human tragedy. The feeling of helplessness, the desire to give up, and the guilt of being unable to help become meaningful when recognized and discussed within the group.

Another type of breakthrough in routine supervisory work came as a result of a series of media articles after a newborn was found left by a garbage bin close to a camp of Ukrainian refugees. As is self-evident, an investigation followed to find the mother. However, the event brought into focus the issue of abortion for refugees and their legal coverage. How protected are employees from law and much more from the debates and criticisms in newspapers and on the Internet in cases of disclosure of some controversial incidents such as unwanted pregnancy, which, by the nature of the refugee situation, are frequent, even between teenagers ?

I met the group of caregivers frozen. Of course, it was one of the times we dealt with their feelings, not with any particular refugee. I think the opportunity to talk immediately about what froze them resulted from the smaller group and the fewer injured refugees they were taking in compared to the group of caregivers on Lesvos.

Most spoke of a sense of loss of meaning in their work and a sense of betrayal after feeling accused. At the same time, there was no room for discussion. From the state they told them to continue their work undisturbed. In the above case and many similar cases, I believe that the possibility of logical explanation is overestimated, and the need to understand the people involved in the irrational and unconscious dimensions of their mental functioning is underestimated.

We discussed Greece's legal system, which cannot be applied to refugees who do not have access to the loopholes that citizens know how to use. The repeal of abortion rights in the United States that overturned the historic 1973 *Roe v. Wade* decision has sparked much debate worldwide. In Greece, abortion was allowed in 1978 in some cases and under certain conditions. What happens to a refugee who does not meet these conditions? Does a private doctor or an NGO undertake to help her in her medical facilities, or is she at risk of legal prosecution? Moreover, if he is not in danger of being prosecuted, is he in danger from the people's courts that have flooded the Internet and acted without a sense of the violence they inflict on those directly involved?

In supervising that day, caregivers said how unfair it is to feel involved in conversations with relatives and friends who "voyeuristically" want to know about the "scandal." The common feeling was that they felt rebellious against the media, but on the other hand, they could not substantiate why they felt they were being blamed. I searched for relevant articles in several newspapers, and there was no accusation against either the carers or the mother. The reporter wrote that the police were looking for the latter for better care.

Once again, the argument for better care could not create the necessary security for caregivers, even more so for refugees. I reflected on this tendency to feel blamed and remembered that in psychoanalysis, when the analyst feels blamed by his analyst, the analyst looks for an unconscious feeling of guilt.

I remembered the case I had read in the *New York Times* about the suicide of a survivor of a tragedy. On October 27, 2023, an article was published (by Choe Sang-Hun, *New York Times*) about the tragedy in Seoul in celebration of Halloween – 153 dead and 83 injured. The journalist wrote that the country's authorities denied responsibility, and the tragedy became a point of political controversy. Most nightmarish, the reporter wrote, was the survivors' sense of guilt for not being able to protect their deceased loved ones. I told the team about the incident, and we talked about the guilt we feel from working in the refugee field, which often leads to confrontation with the NGO management, the state, or the supervisor.

The third incision took place with an e-mail, in which I was asked to bring with me articles talking about ending treatment. Such a move had never happened before, and I was worried. What were they asking for? What articles should I think of about ending treatment when I did not know why I was being asked for them? When I arrived unprepared and troubled, they told me that they had been told that the government closes this particular program for the refugees in Athens because it needs its forces to help with the destruction taking place elsewhere in Greece (catastrophic fires due to climatic change).

What can one say in such a case? The scale of the disaster exceeds any individuality. However, we were already quite "close." I told them that together, we would "write" the chapter for the end. We did not need to read articles. We needed to stay together and get close to what we felt. It was the first time I felt the ambivalence of the team. The aggression and questioning were intense. They told me in many ways that they were not psychoanalysts and did not have the "luxury" of this approach.

For a while, I felt inside me once again the discomfort of dealing with refugees, the thought that it is a masochistic element of my personality that I have not sufficiently analyzed, an unconscious guilt to abandon my ancestors who have suffered from refugee, war, and death. And then, as usual, I remembered my analyst, my supervisors, the welcome of aggression in a relationship of mutual trust and love. There was a moment of rupture inside me, a war, which showed how much we were at war at that moment, in the room of our conversation in Athens, in Gaza, in the world.

I remembered a correctional officer who said you can put a rabid dog in a cage, but he would not want to be in front when you open the door (Gilligan 1996). So, I felt no need to imprison our anger, disappointment, and feeling of eradication. We can all become rabid dogs when faced with something traumatic, especially in circumstances that have increased our vulnerability. However, we can also strengthen our connection in moments of disconnection. I remained silent once more, exploring my experience.

Next time, the team continued with what we had achieved so far in this supervision and what we could still offer. Even if they didn't have the time or desire to write an article as we considered it, they talked about how much they learned that enriched their way of working and how to be in their relationships – with others and with themselves.

When I was writing it, I thought that somewhere here I could see the third principle mentioned by Leuzinger-Bohleber and which I consider particularly important: the exit from passivity through being enraged as the only psychic reaction to an active attitude that allows the powers of love, strength, and resiliency of all to be recovered and strengthened.

Elements of Theory

Psychoanalysts who conceive of man primarily as a participant in a network of relationships, such as relational psychoanalysts, consider the establishment and maintenance of a sense of identity and self to be the hierarchically superior pursuit of man. At the level of the subject interested in psychoanalysis, identity is an experience of internal continuity in change.

Refugees have lost the space (otherwise the field) where they belong and where they have created their capital (cultural, social, and economic) (Bourdieu and Passeron 1990; Prieur and Sestoft 2006). Cultural, social, economic, and symbolic capital, an important part of their identity, determine their place in the social fabric. Therefore, at the same time, the refugee journey has destroyed the sense of belonging to a social fabric.

Identity is a concept that psychoanalysts have avoided, following the attitude of Freud himself, who only used this word once in his extensive work. Avoidance, obviously, not by chance. The concept of identity orients us to characterizations that place the subject within a group (I am Greek, I am socialist, I am a Christian, I am homosexual, I am a man, I am a woman, etc.). The above "identities" are considered external to the internal experience of the person concerned by psychoanalysis but also often unstable and easily alternate, so it is considered that dealing with the concept of identity would unnecessarily complicate the psychoanalytic perspective. Or maybe not?

The need to internalize secure ways of relating to the other (where basic trust in the other has collapsed) can facilitate the integration of the extremely traumatized person into networks of relationships (where the rupture of the family and social fabric has usually contributed to flight) and is a therapeutic goal about which psychoanalytic thinking has much to say (Schottenbauer et al. 2008).

What matters in the refugee field, where there have been catastrophic ruptures in the social fabric, is rediscovering a sense of belonging and continuity despite the constant disasters. Although the immediate needs after trauma are pressing, when there is the possibility of a longer-term intervention, the goal of the therapy goes from the reestablishment of the mentalizing process to the understanding of the more complex object-relational mechanisms and dynamics (Christopoulou et al. 2023).

The axis of transfer and countertransference, which is a central field of interest of psychoanalysis, is offered for the search of the refugee's experience (detecting his experience via the experience of the carer), the reality of the event that stigmatized him, and the rupture in his until then continuous and often coherent biography. Of course, modifications of classical psychoanalytic technique are indicated, given the particularly traumatic nature of the refugee experience. Moreover, transference and countertransference developments often take specific forms such as nonverbal, bodily manifestations, and enactments (Luci and Kahn 2021; Varvin 2019).

In any case, creating a containing environment may facilitate the avoidance of toxic narratives (Linenthal 2001). Toxic narratives are the ones that, emphasizing the traumatic event and its sometimes religious or political messages, become personally empty.

Insistence on closeness in demanding situations heals by offering the security of nonabandonment and nonbetrayal. In war, if there is no faith in help from the comrade-in-arms, nothing is left but chaos and abandonment of battle. Claude Barrois argues that every victim of extreme trauma embodies the rupture of the social fabric:

> Nothing in modern civilization is offered that can help reintegrate the victim into the world of the living. Psychoanalysis has the merit of being the only discipline that actually does something. He rediscovers

the trace of a point of rupture and a "before" where fantasy and dream had their place. Because death, the death that one saw in the face, has no representation.

(Barrois in Briole et al. 1994, 73)

I referred to the principles cited by Dr Leuzinger-Bohleber. Several years ago, before World War I, physician Thomas Salmon also formulated some principles that became the heart of frontline psychiatry, forward psychiatry.
    I will quote at this point the principles of Salmon:

Proximity: opens up a new area of credibility in the face of chaos. Immediacy: a living temporality in contact with the urgent.Expectancy: build a slot after returning from hell.Simplicity: the necessity to raise the subject without idiosyncrasy.

(Davoine and Gaudilliere 2004, 211)

Having heard these principles many years ago, I would like to deliver them to the next ones as they emerged in this complex field of refugees and their caregivers. Most of the caregivers we worked with came to talk about their personal affairs, invited me to work with them at the next refugee camp where they have gone, or later on came for training at the Hellenic Psychoanalytic Society. Unfortunately, I have been forced to refuse often because I am alone. At other times, I have not even been able to answer because of the workload of the moment, which fills me with remorse. All I can do for those whom I have not been able to meet their needs is write this book – and I dedicate it to them.

Bibliography

Barrois, C. 1994. In Le *traumatisme psychique: rencontre et devenir*, edited by Guy Briole, François Lebigot, Bernard Lafont et al. Paris: Masson.

Boulanger, G. 2007. *Wounded by Reality: Understanding and Treating Adult-Onset Trauma*, 180. Mahwah: The Analytic Press.

Bourdieu, Pierre, and Jean-Claude Passeron. 1990. *Reproduction in Education, Society and Culture*. Translated by Richard Nice. 2nd ed. London: SAGE Publications.

Briole, G., F. Lebigot, B. Lafont, J-D. Favre, and D. et Vallet. 1994. *Le traumatisme psychique: rencontre et devenir. Congres de psychiatrie et de neurologie de langue francaise*. Paris: Masson.

Christopoulou, Anna L., Chrysi Giannoulaki, and Nikolaos Tzavaras. 2022. "Mourning and Issues of Identity in the Treatment of Refugees in Lesvos." In *Trauma, Flight and Migration: Psychoanalytic Perspectives*, edited by Anna L. Christopoulou, Chrysi Giannoulaki, and Nicholas Tzavaras, 13–30. London and New York: Routledge.

Davoine, Gaudilliere, Françoise Davoine, and Jean-Max Gaudilliére. 2004. *History Beyond Trauma: Whereof One Cannot Speak, Thereof One Cannot Stay Silent*. Translated by Susan Fairfield, 211. New York: Other Press.

Devereux, Georges. 2015. *Essays on Ethnopsychoanalysis*. Translated into Greek Terzakis, Fotis. Trikala: Epekeina Publications.

Doctors of the World. 2021a. "SYRIA." Accessed July 1, 2021. https://doctorsoftheworld.org/project/Syria/.

Doctors of the World. 2021b. "Greece." Accessed July 1, 2021. https://doctorsoftheworld.org/project/Greece/.

Giannoulaki, C. (2023). Is psychoanalysis of any help for refugees? In Trauma, Flight and Migration, Edited by Vivienne Elton et al. Psychoanalytic Perspectives. Routledge.

Gilligan, J. (1996). Violence: Reflections on a national epidemic. Ed: Vintage Publishing or Knopf Doubleday Publishing Group.

Leuzinger-Bohleber, M. 2021. "Top Authors Project Video Collection." *PEP/UCL* 1 (1): 35.

Leuzinger-Bohleber, M. et al. (2016). What can psychoanalysis contribute to the current refugee crisis? Preliminary reports from STEP-BY-STEP: A psychoanalytic pilot project for supporting refugees in a "First reception camp" and crisis intervention with traumatized refugees. *International Journal of Psychoanalysis*. 97: 1077–1093.

Linenthal, E.T. 2001. *The Unfinished Bombing: Oklahoma City in American Memory.* New York: Oxford University Press.

Luci, M., and M. Kahn. 2021. "Analytic Therapy with Refugees: Between Silence and Embodied Narratives." *Psychoanalytic Inquiry* 41: 103–14.

Marrus, Michael. 1985. *The Unwanted: European Refugees in the Twentieth Century.* USA: Oxford University Press.

Papadopoulos, Renos. 2019. *Psychosocial Dimensions of the Refugee Condition – A Synergistic Approach.* Athens: Babel Day Center/Syn-eirmos NGO of Social Solidarity & the Centre for Trauma, Asylum and Refugees of the University of Essex.

Prieur, Annick, and Carsten Sestoft. 2006. *Pierre Bourdieu: En introduktion.* Copenhagen: Hans Reitzels Forlag.

Seeley, K. 2005. "Trauma as Metaphor: The Politics of Psychotherapy After September 11, 2001." *Psychotherapy and Politics International* 3: 17–27.

Schottenbauer, Michele A. et al. 2008. "Nonresponse and Dropout Rates in Outcome Studies on PTSD: Review and Methodological Considerations." *Psychiatry: Interpersonal and Biological Processes* 71 (2): 134–68.

Varvin, S. 2019. "Psychoanalysis and the Situation of Refugees: A Human Rights Perspective." In *Psychoanalysis, Law and Society*, edited by P. Montagna and A. Harris, 9–26. New York: Routledge and Taylor and Francis Group.

Varvin, S. 2023. "Psychoanalysis and the Third Position: Social Upheavals and Atrocity." *The International Journal of Psychoanalysis* 104 (3): 574–84.

11 Countertransference and Xenos

The Question

In 2024, fear of and aggression toward refugees and migrants met with an unprecedented escalation worldwide – in the United States, they contributed to the reelection of former president Donald Trump. Characteristically, in a *New York Times* article titled "Xenophobia and Hate Speech Are Spiking Heading into the Election," Yonatan Lupu, an associate professor of political science at George Washington University, stressed: "I certainly do not remember in my lifetime the rhetoric against immigrants ever getting this strong during an election" (Amy Qin 2024).

The intense xenophobia with which we react to refugees has its source in fear of the "Xenos." Xenos in ancient Greek means the Other, the outsider, the visitor, the wanderer. Moreover, Xenos is also sacred. In ancient Greece, the father of the gods, Zeus, had the epithet Xenios, emphasizing that Zeus protects any wanderer or refugee person (who is not a robber or enemy) by imposing the sacred duty to protect and care for them (Liddell and Scott 2007).

Ambivalence toward the stranger caught Freud's attention, particularly in the text Das Unheimlich (1919). In the preceding chapters, we have dealt with nostalgia. Heimweh in German is nostalgia for one's homeland, heimat is homeland, and heim is, broadly, home. In the above text, Freud states that the uncanny is a form of the frightening, which goes back to something already known and familiar. "The uncanny is that class of the frightening which leads back to what is known of old and long familiar" (Freud 1919, 220). Freud points out its ambiguity: "Thus Heimlich is a word whose meaning develops in the direction of ambivalence until it finally coincides with its opposite, unheimlich. Unheimlich is in some way or other a subspecies of Heimlich" (Freud 1919, 226).

Ambivalence toward refugees is one of the main characteristics of the affects in the caring person and/or the group, thus a trait of the countertransference in the psychoanalytic glossary. We can see the ambivalence in both the consulting room and the society. In the former, the encounter with the refugee is filled with gross countertransference problems. In the latter, society neglects the refugees' present situation, thus denying the necessary

DOI: 10.4324/9781003639022-12

acknowledgment of the trauma and the assignment of meaning to trau-matizing experiences, which is a prerequisite for the rehabilitation of the refugees.

In the second chapter of *The Uncanny*, Freud mentions as the most appro-priate case of the uncanny, the "doubts whether an inanimate being is gen-uinely alive; or conversely, a lifeless object might not be really animate" (Freud 1919, 226). Terror, aggression, and admiration for the nonliving, the inanimate, meet in Kohut's *Thoughts on Narcissism and Narcissistic Rage* (1972): "Apprehensions about the aliveness of self and body and the repu-diation of these fears by the assertion that the animate can yet be graceful, even perfect" (Kohut 1972, 361).

In Kafka's novel *Metamorphosis*, Gregor is faced with something unthink-able for a man to happen to him, but is *the unthinkable* as rare as we would like to believe? Or is it too well known to us, too familiar in a particular way, as Freud stated in *The Uncanny*?

We are all refugees and strangers as we are born on a coastline between the mythical way of being before the consciousness of self and object and the world of reality. Man seeks to procure unity to the perception of himself in a world of constant change; in other words, he seeks a sense of personal identity. Erikson (1956) theorized as a "sense of identity" the existence of conviction (and not just an impulse, desire, or will) and self-confidence (confidence in oneself, not merely satiety, satisfaction, or happiness).

The identity that man wants to think of as unified can regress to be felt fragmented or even lost. The refugees' trauma is dehumanizing. The loss of humanity and the ineffable anguish and loneliness that follow are of particular interest to refugees' carers. The concept of metamorphosis, that is of transforming the animate into the inanimate, is an appropriate meta-phor for the state of a part of the psyche that has lost (in conditions where a person is confronted with something that does not fit the human mind) the human identity and, therefore, the ability to speak and reflect (Giannoulaki 2023, forthcoming).

Adriana Prengler, at the IPA webinar on "Refugees and Immigrants: How Can Psychoanalysis Contribute?" highlights the importance of lan-guage in the constant classification of someone as a "Xenos." Even if the refugee or migrant learns the language, his pronunciation will make him a stranger in every sentence and every word he pronounces.

Prengler, who herself was an immigrant – she immigrated to the United States in 2010 and was chair of the IPA's Psychoanalysts' Emigration and Relocation Committee (PERC) – insisted, among other things, on the importance of losing the sense of identity and belonging. "Immigration is a complex process involving the loss of feelings of identity and belonging among many losses. There is the feeling of becoming a stranger to others and us" (Prengler 2019).

He who does not speak our language is, by definition, Xenos. We are all Xenos coming to the world, as we do not have the possibility to understand

and be understood via words. However, symbolic mediation concerns symbols on all levels, not only verbal high-level but also bodily signs and gestures, which are of extreme value in the mother–newborn dyad. The infant internalizes the semiotic universe of the mother–infant dyad and creates the possibility for different levels of mentalization, including bodily expression, acting, dreaming, and higher levels of abstraction.

Words and language remain the principal medium through which we construct links between the body and the psychic. According to Freudian theory, unmetalized experiences, "raw" experiences, are channeled into mental content via word representations. This is why researchers on trauma conclude that listening to refugees requires the psychoanalyst's attunement to process and content in each individual's accounts of the past and to unsymbolized pieces of affect that are transmitted intersubjectively (Auerhan 2023).

Speaking of "strange" feelings and self, states that cannot be put into words, and their "refugee journey" within ourselves, I find it interesting that Greek physicians and philosophers of the fourth century BC described hysterical symptoms as consequences of the journey, of wandering, of the "*ystera*" in the body (*ystera* is the uterus in ancient Greek):

> in women ... the uterus ... a living being within them has the desire to procreate, and if this desire is not fulfilled at the right time, he becomes aggrieved and angry and wanders throughout the body... and causes all kinds of disturbances.
>
> (Plato, Timaeus)

The observation of the existence of foreign and angry elements of the body wandering within it, the functioning of the uterus and menstruation, and its consequences on the perfusion of the brain brought Hippocrates, to whom Hysteria is attributed, *close to modern neurobiological research* (Buchan 1999; King 1998).

Van Der Kolk writes about speechless horror that correlates it with Broca's area, which is the brain's center for speech. Without a functioning Broca's area, you cannot put your thoughts and feelings into words. The scans showed that Broca's area went offline whenever a flashback was triggered (Van Der Kolk 2014, 43).

Through special interest in the unconscious, psychoanalytic theory and clinical practice have shown that our unconscious speaks in a different language than we do not understand. We must interpret work to understand our unconscious images of a dream, the meaning of one lapsus, etc.

The interpretation of the refugees' words, behavior, and suffering also needs an "interpretation" to be put into words and to acquire meaning. "When individuals are caught up in a catastrophically overwhelming event, inducing total helplessness, their sudden enforced regression takes them back to a stage before the use of words and symbolic thinking have emerged in their development" (Garland 1998, 120).

The word does not represent the event; it is the event. The word is not a symbol for the thing but the thing itself. Consequently, the question of whether the triggering of memory can potentially bring about the explosion of an uncontrollable and lethal stimulation that cannot be associated with any representation or word and that no one can fit and metabolize (Donnet 2009) is crucial.

In case the psychoanalyst tries to get in contact with the pre-traumatic personality of the patient, the refugee thinks perhaps that his experience of the trauma is too challenging to be recognized by the other (Bergmann 1998). He can become silent, withdraw, and discontinue the treatment as the way he experiences himself as a consequence of trauma can be described in simple words: nothing will be exactly as it was before.

The descent into Hades is not a random image. A mythological reference (apart from the image of the living dead) is Orpheus, who, returning from Hades, no longer sings. The survivors of a tragedy return from the place of the dead, and the therapist is called upon to decipher the untimely images, the fossilized experiences that the victims are unable to recognize and narrate. Instead, they trace and present them without recognizing or feeling them (Davoine and Gaudilliere 2004, 209).

On the other hand, the transition from the traumatic area where the refugee is stuck with the trauma as the dominating feature of mental life to an ordinary place where he can integrate the traumatic event and begin mourning the loss of the pre-traumatic self and life is possible according to the psychoanalysts who work with traumatized people. It is not about a cathartic release. Instead, the treatment aims to help the process of mourning unfold.

This book aims at and desires to help the therapist endure the agony that enters the axis of transference and countertransference, the ineffable pain, and the cry of the suffering subject without going so far as to show the patient the exit from the analytical relationship as non-analyzable. The desire, thinking on the countertransference's dead ends, is not to bypass the unfolding of the therapeutic possibilities of psychodynamic understanding and therapeutic encounters with the refugee (Varvin 2013, 2016).

In this chapter, I will highlight that in her attempt to save Dahlia, the Ukrainian teenager, the therapist was "saved" herself. I will quote the clinical material and clarify how I mean "saved."

I shall, therefore, talk about Dahlia, a 13-year-old teenager from Ukraine who was lucky enough that her therapist in the refugee camp offered her psychotherapy at a rate of one to three times a week for two and a half years.

Clinical Case

Dahlia is a 14-year-old Ukrainian teenager who came with her family to Greece in March 2022, a month after the Russian invasion of her homeland.

Within two days, the refugee camp where the therapist had been working for the past two years was transformed into a shelter for Ukrainian war refugees.

For the therapist (let's call her Maria), the images she only saw on TV of uprooted people suddenly came too close to her. When Ukrainian mothers with children began to arrive at the camp, as their dress and behavior were close to the image she had of herself and her 3-year-old child, they disturbed her profoundly.

> Maria: These women, especially mothers, are like me; I could be in their place, alone with a child on an unknown journey with many dangers and an unknown destination. Initially, I doubted I could do anything to help them. Gradually, among the tragic stories, I also heard stories that made me think that uprooting for some could also become salvation.

One of those stories that made her think there was a possibility of a happy outcome concerned Dahlia, who went to her at the urging of a friend.

Dahlia's appearance was reminiscent of a boy because of the haircut and dress. She was extremely shy. Dahlia told Maria that her problems are very serious and that she may need a doctor. She raised the point from the outset that she might not be welcome, that she was not in the "right place." So, she was a stranger, a xenos.

Over the past year, the teenager added, her sleep has been completely erratic and intermittent, lasting less than 6 hours around the clock. While in Ukraine, she had made two suicide attempts, the last one three months ago. The parents' attitude was that her problems would improve as she got older and that, for now, she had to find a way to manage them.

The therapist, after meeting with her parents and referring her to the child psychiatrist, prescribed psychotherapy with the frequency of once a week, which after three months was done twice a week and soon three times a week. The practitioner's time at the camp allowed for this frequency – and the interest of both of them in their meetings was great.

Maria asked me to supervise her case with Dahlia, temporarily leaving the rest of the patients she was treating in her office privately. Despite the difficulty of working outside the usual framework, I accepted because my interest was also great.

How would psychodynamic treatment develop with a suicidal teenager, complicated by the trauma of war and refugee? Could the treatment so early in the adolescent's entry into the country offer an alternative to acting outs, such as suicide attempt or recourse to alcohol and delinquent behavior that Dahlia had already expressed during her stay in Ukraine? Or, was it foolhardy and potentially dangerous to cause an uncontrollable regression in a fragile adolescent psyche even before the war and the refugee?

In the first six months, Dahlia was punctual and did not miss any sessions. I will mention some elements from the first period, during which Dahlia developed a very intense transference.

In the seventh session, the therapeutic alliance was established. Dahlia was trustful enough to talk about an inner voice, presenting it as a "friend" she has had since she was young and to whom she has been talking often. She recognized that the voice did not exist as a separate person but nevertheless she experienced it as different from her. Dahlia added that she tries to talk with this friend, especially when she cannot face reality.

When the therapist told her that maybe together, they can face reality, Dahlia replied: "Being together seems strange to me, I am not used to it. However, my friend must also give his permission for us to be together."

In the eighth session, the first verbalization of traumatic memories took place. Dahlia cited an incident of harassment in Ukraine when she was just 8 years old. She added that the most important thing for her at the time was the loss of her cat, with whom she had begun to bond. Maria thought that Dahlia wanted to deny her feelings generated by the harassment and at the same time confess how important it is for her not to lose the beloved object: the cat or Maria. Dahlia had begun to bond with her, and it was difficult for her to separate, especially at the weekend.

In the ninth session, Dahlia reported even more intense reactions to the loss of meetings with Maria.

Dahlia: "Sometimes it is as if I forget faces and who I am. Yesterday, I tried to remember your face, but I could not. I get something like panic attacks at that moment." With Maria's help, Dahlia developed the ability to observe herself, as shown by the excerpts of the sessions.

Tenth Session

Dahlia: Sometimes I feel tension and do not know what to do. I try to cry, but I cannot. What I do is deaden myself for a few minutes, and I feel like nothing is affecting me. I counted the days until I arrived. I had a dream about my cat: it came out from a picture held by a man, and he showed it to me. When he came out of there, I hugged him. My relatives and the person who showed me the picture wanted to prevent me from being with the cat, but I was holding him and running.

The therapist interpreted it as a vivid reflection of Dahlia's feelings and thoughts stirred through their encounters. Dahlia denied this, saying she did not notice any difference in how she felt. Soon after, however, he began to talk about some platonic homosexual relationships in which she did not feel the girl's interest. The one girl she was in love with rejected her. Maria recognized the erotic transfer to which she was responding with an erotic countertransference, as she revealed to me in retrospect. Unfortunately, at this point, there was a sudden 3-week interruption of treatment due to an accident in the therapist's child.

On Maria's return, things had changed. There followed a period of intense mistrust, resistance, and acting out.

> Dahlia: I took some notes while you were away about things I wanted to discuss. I do not know if you heard about my brother being hospitalized because of appendicitis. I was surprised that I was not upset at all. I even joked to the point that my stressed mother got angry. When my mother is done with other people's needs, she needs a reminder to deal with mine, but she still doesn't do it because she feels tired. I just do not care. I am not sorry at all. I have been writing lyrics for the last few years, but I feel like they are not perfected. I describe what I feel, but in a way that if someone reads them, they do not quite understand my experiences, but they can identify with what they are reading.

The therapist did not associate Dahlia's feelings with her absence. We discussed it during supervision. At the next meeting, a painful surprise awaited her.

> Dahlia: I have something interesting to discuss today (she smiled). On Friday night, I made a suicide attempt (she showed her hand). I thought I was going to be stressed or scared but I was just sitting in the bathroom, blood was flowing, and I was waiting for it to happen. I don't know how to manage these thoughts. Suddenly, I felt an overload after repeated events. I feel ashamed that I didn't cut it deeper so that it ended. On the other hand, I think that there are things pending and that there are friends who are interested in me. But I wanted to be selfish, not to care about the people who would lose me.

The therapist's reaction, because of her reduced mental availability at the time, was aggressive because she felt that Dahlia's suicide attempt was an aggressive and manipulative move.

Only, after we discussed that in the supervision, Maria was able to get back into the relationship, saying, "I think you might want me to feel the load you felt when you suddenly lost me."

Dahlia said she had learned why the therapist was absent from an employee at the camp. The connection with the mother, who was anxious about her younger brother's health, was evident.

To help Dahlia and the therapist both process their great anger, I suggested that she ask Dahlia to paint either in the session or in between and talk about the drawings, inspired by Benedetti's use of these techniques.

Although the classical psychoanalytic thesis is that in adolescence painting does not need to be used, bypassing the difficulty of a foreign language and adopting the language of art may have been unifying for the two of them.

With many attacks in the therapeutic framework, since Dahlia often did not go, remaining defiantly in the courtyard of the camp from where the practitioner could see her, the treatment continued.

During the seventh month of treatment, Dahlia brought a painting of herself that she had just made. Her paintings often depict eyes. In this painting, one face is shown in profile. The picture has three eyes. In both eyes, there were many small eyes inside, and the third eye was in the position where the mouth normally is. Something like blood flowed from the third eye. In Greek, there is the expression, *"I eat the other with my eyes."*

Having discussed positivity as a proposal from Benedetti, the therapist tells Dahlia that the eyes do not see, flooded with as many small eyes as tears. However, the mouth sees and, perhaps, cries with tears like blood. Dahlia replies: "I don't know if I can look at the other person. Nor should I speak. I may express my need, and the other person will tell me they are not interested and push me away."

On one occasion, when Dahlia provocatively said that she tore the drawing because nothing made sense, Maria found herself pressing the pencil so hard against the paper that she pierced it. Only then did she realize how much Dahlia was angry at her.

My surprise at this realization from Maria was great because I saw in front of me the change of the supervised therapist I knew, who was a very attentive practitioner, who hardly allowed herself and me to recognize the unconscious behind and below the conscious.

At one point, Maria told me that Dahlia had helped her move forward with her personal therapy like no one before and that only now did she realize how much she herself had not experienced her adolescence.

I thought that, alongside Dahlia, Maria was maturing. Therefore, I was not surprised when Maria, after a year and a half of treating Dahlia, asked me after intense hesitation for my consent to tell at the supervision a dream with Dahlia:

> I saw in a dream that Dahlia addressed a colleague and friend of mine. I felt betrayed by Dahlia. She sold me out at the first opportunity. In the dream, I thought this was because I could not understand and help her.

Listening to her dream, I also thought I was in front of material on at least three levels of relationship: Dahlia's relationship with Maria, Maria's relationship with her analyst, and Maria's relationship with me.

Then, when she hesitated, too agitated to share her associations, I remembered my supervisor's (who was Jean Max Gaudilliere) words, reassuring me when I cried at the supervision without understanding why I was crying, saying, "This is part of our job."

His words pushed me, many years ago, to perceive the place of my encounter with this particular analysand as a place of inner evolution and change not only for her but also for me. I discovered a hidden part of my biography that turned out to be part of the biography of my mother and grandmother.

I said the same words to the therapist: "This is part of our job."

In the supervision, we talked about the countertransferential feelings of guilt and helplessness that the attempt at suicide created in Maria. Maria was able to think about incidents in her biography where her love was hidden by the feelings of guilt and helplessness.

There began a third period of their therapeutic relationship. Now, Maria was the one permitting herself to do acting outs, but not catastrophic ones. On the contrary, she could not help herself putting an end in her desire to "adopt" Dahlia.

For example, she bought a cheap guitar so Dahlia could learn to play music. Dahlia went to guitar lessons and English lessons. She read Machiavelli, and they discussed her readings. Maria admired her for her intelligence and sensitivity, although they often faced ruptures. However, their love was, I think, apparent for both.

Maria's manager at the camp urged her to abandon Dahlia's treatment and Dahlia as unsuitable for psychodynamic approach but she did not obey.

Dahlia's treatment lasted another year and stopped when Maria's work at the camp ended.

After the end of Dahlia's treatment, while Maria expressed her sadness for abandoning her, I was thinking of writing about this therapy. I had a dream that I considered to be part of this work. In the dream, I had to flee an area of danger and war. Then, I noticed one of my analysands I talked about in the supervision with Jean Max Gaudilliere, I referred above. I grabbed her by the hand, as children do to dive from a pier into the sea. We dived into a river that led us away from danger.

This was a dream that I consider to be a positivization of Dahlia's therapist's dream. I was not asked to leave my analysand, just as I did not urge Maria to leave Dahlia. By saving the patient, the therapist can also be saved. The exit from the psychic landscape of death-like stillness is through the "game of speech" created by the two of them.

Elements of Theory

Maria was touched by the case of Dahlia. Did I have to advise her in supervision that such a strong countertransference was a reason not to undertake Dahlia's treatment? Is it possible for someone to undertake the psychodynamic treatment of a refugee, especially a teenager feeling a strong countertransference which will lead to repeated acting outs?

Varvin, who has dealt with similar phenomena in extreme trauma, argues that the injured person, from the beginning of treatment, will confront the analyst with non-symbolized unconscious relationships, which were either stirred, reinforced, or created as a consequence of the trauma in his psyche and which he tries to "show" to the analyst if he cannot talk about them. This will be followed by acting out that includes important aspects of the trauma, which much later will be incorporated into a narrative (Varvin 2013).

In general, pathological conditions that translate experiences of mental death of the patient are recognized as having the ability to force the analyst's unconscious to move out of the landscape of mental death and immobility, regardless of his logic, will, or mental formation. These movements appear in night dreams or in daytime fantasies.

Maria was gripped by fantasies about adopting Dahlia, which she feared had driven her away from caring for her child. Her guilt led her to talk a lot about Dahlia, and her manager was also alarmed. One could, of course, interpret her countertransference as a narcissistic defensive psychic move, an idealization of herself, stemming from her guilt in abandoning her depressed mother to intrapsychic reality.

The manager was partly right, but by abandoning her depressed mother, Maria would also abandon her creative, childish, and adolescent self, "devoured" by the traumatized self that was driven too early to a false maturity. Maria had become a psychologist to revive her mother and herself. Dahlia was her chance to make big progress toward her true self.

Often, a reaction of the therapist takes place that can be considered as a countertransferential acting out (Jacobs 1986) which, however, is a starting point of communication between therapist and patient, a starting point of a relationship, despite the climate of mistrust and fear resulting from the core mental destruction of the victim.

In Dahlia's case, telling her (Dahlia's) story allowed Maria to connect disconnected aspects of herself. In some modern conceptions of the psyche, the unconscious includes not only the repressed but also that which has not yet been formulated, has not taken a form, and, therefore, has not been expressed. Based on the above position, we are not looking for a revelation of psychic contents that had already been formed and repelled but rather to give form to what has no form and, through words, to articulate what has not been articulated verbally. However, an experience not yet schematized must be coconstructed in interaction with someone else, in this case, the therapist for Dahlia and Dahlia for the therapist.

Understanding results from the interaction of the analyst's and analysand's experiences creates the intersubjective dimension of the psychoanalytic encounter. The possibility, through the interpretative work of the psychoanalyst, of bringing about change in the psyches of both the analysand and the analyst raises again the limits of language and its relationship with human nature and culture.

By broadening the term countertransference and outside the psycho-analytic framework, I could argue that the xenophobic attitude is the con-sequence of the "countertransference" of each person, the reaction of his psyche to the entry of the extreme traumatic rupture into his daily life. Consequently, a desire to restore the former equilibrium is created, accom-panied by the desire to destroy the foreign element. The refugee is equated with what he carries; he becomes the symbol of the catastrophe that, if we destroy it, we will be relieved of the pain of his sense of identity rupture.

Images of terrorist attacks by foreigners quickly surface at the slightest detection of violence, aggression, and a desire for revenge on the part of refugees. Moreover, because of the tendency for repetition of trauma that Freud has pointed out and has been observed by experts in various fields of science dealing with traumatized people, the behavior of most trauma-tized subjects does not reinforce the constant desire over time to help them. Pushing to the extreme the psychoanalytic thesis that a human defense is to actively do what he suffers passively, those who defend the protection of borders against the influx of refugees invoke it as an argument: Those who have been victims of extreme trauma will be the future perpetrators of extreme violent attacks, such as terrorist attacks.

Marianne Leuzinger-Bohleber and Sverre Varvin, at the IPA webinar on "Refugees and Immigrants: How Can Psychoanalysis Contribute?", described this argument as a mythical generalization. I would argue that even when we adopt this way of thinking, we become fundamentalists ourselves because totalitarian thinking makes things one-dimensional and destroys the possibilities of transforming meaning.

Meeting a patient potentially promises a space of freedom and creativity. The need to recognize and encourage the creative side of the refugee therapist's mental work plays an important role in the refugee's treatment and/or supervision. As in Maria's case, this can open the way to the thera-pist's analysis at the same time as the evolution of the refugee's treatment, here Dahlia.

"When speech stops, a new language game must be invented" is a well-known saying of Wittgenstein. In simpler words, in order for someone to speak, his speech must be set in motion in an atmosphere of creating a new way of communicating in order to get out of the stillness where he enters moments of extreme trauma.

The psychoanalyst's psyche, in critical phases during his work (con-sciously, preconsciously, or unconsciously), when he enters a field of men-tal destruction, undertakes to create some vehicle of signification of what happens in the encounter with the injured patient. The emergence of emo-tions, dream fantasies, and daydreams within the psyche is an unconscious choice. Therefore, the analyst needs to focus on these formations (attention is a conscious choice).

What takes place within the analyst's psyche is externalized; that is, it reaches his consciousness through various and different symbolic forms.

The refuge (in the sense that the analyst's thinking finds refuge in this form of thinking in conditions difficult for his psyche) and the emergence of each form is, of course, part of the countertransference. Ernst Cassirer, in *his Philosophy of Symbolic Forms*, argues intelligibly:

> The human spirit only ends up externalizing its true and perfect inwardness. The form in which the innermost manifests determines and retrospectively its nature and content.... It does not simply depict or mirror the experience; it gives it a specific form and physiognomy, which, in its first, repeatable realization, in turn, has a formative effect on the inner life itself.
>
> (Eilenberger 2018, 155)

The use of the painting technique and positivity in interpretation is from Benedetti's books (1995, 1998) as I understood them through the supervision I did with my supervisors Davoine, F. and Gaudilliere, J.-M. Their theory and clinic of trauma and its intergenerational transmission are included in their books, especially *Histoire et Trauma* (2004). The emphasis on countertransference and on technique as means to help the patient integrate warded off self-aspects does not disempower the connection between trauma and real social catastrophes. Treatment and rehabilitation approaches need to take social and cultural conditions into consideration as the majority of the refugees are not so lucky as Dahlia and continue to live under difficult conditions in refugee camps and shelters. But an understanding on how traumatic experience is actualized in the transference and bring the analyst in a situation where enactments inevitably occur can encourage further research. The aim of the treatment remains

> for the traumatic event to become part of the survivor's overall thinking and functioning, instead of remaining a split-off, encapsulated and avoided area, a "foreign body" in the mind, ready to break open once more at the next unforeseen and frightening incident.
>
> (Garland 1998, 122)

Bibliography

Auerhan, N. 2023. "I Can't Forget What You Couldn't Tell Me: A Psychoanalyst Listens to Asylum Seekers." *The Psychoanalytic Quarterly* 92: 185–221. https://doi.org/10.1080/00332828.2023.2237507.

Benedetti, G. 1995. *La mort dans l'âme*. Translated by P. Faugeras Ramonville-Sainte-Agne. Paris: Erès.

Benedetti, G. 1998. *Le sujet emprunté*. Translated by P. Faugeras. Ramonville-Sainte-Agne, Paris: Erès.

Bergmann, M. S. 1998. "Die Interaktion zwischen Trauma und intrapsychischem Konflikt in der Geschichte der Psychoanalyse." In *Trauma Und Konflikt*, edited by A-M. Schlösser and K. Höhfeld, 113–30. Giessen: Psychosozial Verlag.

Buchan Morag. (1999). *Women in Plato's political theory*. London; Ed. Macmillan Press LTD.

Davoine, F., and J.-M. Gaudilliere. 2004. "Histoire et Trauma." In *Greek. History and Trauma (2013)*, translated by Marina Kounezis, edited by Yiannis Gkiastas. Methexis.

Donnet, J. L. 2009. *The Analyzing Situation*. Translated by Andrew Weller. London: Karnac.

Eilenberger, W. 2018. *The Age of the Magi: The Great Ten Years of Philosophy 1919–1929*. Translated by Koilis Giannis. Athens: Patakis Publications.

Erikson, E. H. 1956. "The Problem of Ego Identity." *Journal of the American Psychoanalytic Association* 4: 56–121.

Erikson, E. H. 1964. "Identity and Uprootedness in Our Time." In *Insight and Responsibility*, edited by Erik H. Erikson, 81–107. New York: Norton.

Freud, S. 1919. "The Uncanny." *Standard Edition* 17: 217–56.

Garland, C. 1998. *Understanding Trauma: A Psychoanalytical Approach*. Edited by Caroline Garland. London: Karnac.

Giannoulaki, C. 2023. "Is Psychoanalysis of Any Help for Refugees?" In *Trauma, Flight and Migration: Psychoanalytic Perspectives*, edited by the series IPA in the Community. London and New York: Routledge.

Jacobs, T. 1986. "On Counter-Transference Enactments." *Journal of the American Psychoanalytic Association* 34: 289–307.

Kafka, F. 1915. *Metamorphosis*. Ell. Edition. Kafka, F. *Metamorphosis (2012)*. Translated by Margarita Zachariadou. Athens: Patakis Publications.

King, Helen. (1998). Hippocrates's women. New York: Routledge.

Kohut, H. 1972. "Thoughts on Narcissism and Narcissistic Rage." *Psychoanalytic Study of the Child* 27: 360–400.

Leuzinger-Bohleber, M. 2019. "Refugees and Immigrants: How Can Psychoanalysis Contribute?" IPA's Webinar.

Lifton, R. J. 1968. *Death in Life: Survivors of Hiroshima*. New York: Random House.

Lifton, R. J. 1972. "On Psychohistory." *Psychoanalysis and Contemporary Science* 1: 355–372.

Lifton, R. J. 1973. "The Sense of Immortality: On Death and the Continuity of Life." *American Journal of Psychoanalysis* 33 (1): 3–15.

Lifton, R. J. 1976. "From Analysis to Formation: Towards a Shift in Psychological Paradigm." *Journal of the American Academy of Psychoanalysis* 4: 63–94.

Liddell, H. G., and R. Scott. 1889. *An Intermediate Greek-English Lexicon*. Translated into Greek (2007) under the title: *The Epitome of the Great Dictionary of the Greek Language*. (2007) Athens: Pelekanos Publications, Oxford: Clarendon Press.

Prengler, A. 2019. "Refugees and Immigrants: How Can Psychoanalysis Contribute?" IPA's Webinar.

Van Der Kolk, B. A., A. C. McFarlane, and L. Weisaeth. 1996. *Traumatic Stress*. New York: Guilford Press.

Van Der Kolk, B. (2014). *The body keeps the score. Brain, Mind and body in the healing of trauma*. USA; Viking Ed.

Varvin, S. 1998. "Psychoanalytic Psychotherapy with Traumatized Refugees: Integration, Symbolization and Mourning." *American Journal of Psychotherapy* 52 (1): 64–71.

Varvin, S. 2003. *Mental Survival Strategies After Extreme Traumatisation*. Copenhagen: Multivers.

Varvin, S. 2013. "Trauma als Nonverbale Kommunikation" (Trauma as Nonverbal Communication). *Zeitschrift für psychoanalytische Theorie und Praxis* 28: 114–30.

Varvin, S. 2016. "Psychoanalysis with the Traumatized Patient: Helping to Survive Extreme Experiences and Complicated Loss." *International Forum of Psychoanalysis* 25 (2): 73–80.

Varvin, S. 2019. "Refugees and Immigrants: How Can Psychoanalysis Contribute?" IPA's Webinar.

Qin, A. November 6, 2024. "Xenophobia and Hate Speech Are Spiking Heading into the Election." *New York Times.*

12 Intergenerational Transmission
Memory and Oblivion

The Question

We use the notion of *Trauma* to refer to "any experience which calls up distressing affects – such as those of fright, anxiety, shame, or physical pain" (Breuer and Freud 1895, 6). In the case of trauma, the protective shield is ruptured – by definition and leaves a mark! Trauma cannot be removed from the mind; it haunts it. Refugees cannot get rid of the trauma that returns repeatedly provoking affects such as frifht, shame and physcal pain in an otherwise unexplicable degree. Trauma is not only the wound left on the skin or the psyche after an injury. It is also a chance for regeneration. Even if ffects generated are hard for the ego to cope with and multiple defensive mechanisms set in motion there is almost always the potential for healing with a good enough strategic treatment

How can one achieve oblivion?

Initially, it seems paradoxical that psychoanalysis, which originally aimed to fill mnemonic gaps, seeks oblivion rather than memory. In classical psychoanalytic literature, the presence or construction of the past in the present experience was considered central from the outset. The past is sought at every moment of the psychoanalytic process (LaFarge 2014; Levine 2009; Scarfone 2006). As the analysis "progresses" through time, "deeper" layers of the psychic apparatus are approached, and experiences and fantasies belonging to various periods of life emerge as transference and countertransference are interweaved. Sometimes, a suicide or a serious mental illness, often toward the psychotic end of the spectrum, or an unexplained force of destruction, can suddenly enter one's analytic relationship – or life – and thus bring the scene of trauma into the present.

In the above paragraph, two forms of *experience recall* are recognized. One is within the realm of speech, the symbolic, and the other beyond it. In other words, the way the past is rewritten into the here and now of a neurotic analysand's therapy is different from the way the nightmare of trauma is experienced repeatedly in a refugee's sleep and wakefulness.

Memory and truth, fantasy in its conscious and unconscious forms, preoccupied Freud from the beginning to the end of his work (Masson 1985). When Freud abandoned his first theory that started from the memories of

DOI: 10.4324/9781003639022-13

hysterical patients, which he accepted as true, he turned to the importance of fantasies over experiences.

(A) The actual events experienced by the child, from the moment he experienced them onward, were considered no less important than their inner narrative. In psychoanalysis, the analysand narrates the same event repeatedly in search of a special meaning to emerge, a particular sense of truth, which in its transparency will surprise him, and he will feel that everything is in place instantaneously. This is the first form of experience recall.

(B) According to the Freudian view, not everyone – or not everyone always – has the ability to narrate their past; some experience it in the Here and Now. Trauma causes many and varied disturbances of Time as a subjective experience. For example, the immobilization of time as a result of a traumatic experience is well known: the trauma remains present "as if it happened yesterday." The freezing of time is accompanied by the fear of a particularly short life and the fear of Death (Kernberg 2008). This is the second form of experience recall.

The need to weaken the defensive reactions of the psyche as a consequence of trauma through the reinforcement of self-observation and speech (in other words, through the strengthening of the symbolic function at the expense of the one-dimensional, timeless domination of a *discours operatoire*), the need to internalize safe ways of relating to the other, the need to integrate the injured person into networks of relationships (where usually the rupture of the family and social fabric has contributed to fleeing), the need to strengthen self-esteem and, last but not least, self-constitution cannot be achieved in one generation and, often, the effects of trauma pass on to subsequent generations. The transgenerational transmission of trauma has been studied by prominent analysts in the realm of adult and child survivors of the Holocaust (Kestenberg 1980; Kestenberg & Brenner 1996; Kestenberg & Kahn 1998; Brenner 2002; Kogan 2002a, 2002b, 2019).

How can trauma be transmitted to the second or even the third generation?

The contemporary psychoanalytic theory holds that

> secrets, unexplained flare-ups of temper, constant transposition of the past on the present, survival anxiety, avoidances of related topics, overprotectiveness towards children combined with covert devaluation of their problems as trivial, and holding up an unrealistically high ideal (for children, that is) of stoicism and resilience contribute to how the trauma can be transmitted to the second or even the third generation.

Many traumatic stories reach the analytical process in the third generation when someone – who can deal with himself – is confronted with inexplicable collapses of time in his life. These inexplicable breaks call him to fight his own battle with the ghosts of the past – a battle for which he asks for the cooperation of the analyst. The analyst is asked to decipher the untimely images. In order to be able to contribute to the therapeutic work, the analyst must be able to perceive for himself the oft-silent appearance of the above phenomena, furthermore bearing in mind that despite the destructiveness that accompany them, they create possibilities for healing. Trauma is a double-edged sword: it can cause fixation and traumatic neurosis, but it can also lead to vigilance, self-protectiveness, perseverance, curiosity, and altruistic tendencies (Akhtar 1995). The outcome of trauma depends, of course, on multiple factors.

Papadopoulos (2002) stresses that in ancient Greek, a more thorough exploration of the word trauma suggests that the root of *titrosko* (τιτρώσκω) is likely to be *τείρω* (tir-o), which means to rub. In ancient Greek, the verb tiro had two opposite meanings, i.e., to rub in and off/away. Based on this, "trauma would be the mark left on people as a result of something being rubbed onto them" (Papadopoulos 2007, 304). So, depending on the different connotations of the verb (tiro), it can be inferred that trauma may involve the meaning of wound or injury as a result of rubbing in, or it may refer to rubbing away the marks on a surface, i.e., the result of erasing or cleansing (Papadopoulos 2002, 2007).

The analyst needs to be able to perceive in the intrapsychic space of the analysand *the* dimension of the appearance of an intergenerational trauma. A reaction of the therapist takes often place that can be considered as a countertransferential acting out (Jacobs 1986) which, however, is a starting point of communication between therapist and patient, a starting point of a relationship. The above acting out is a bridge that is constructed besides the climate of mistrust and fear resulting from the core mental destruction of the victim. These acting outs include important aspects of trauma, which will be integrated into a narrative much later (Varvin 2013).

As a technique proposal, it is recommended that the analyst identify peculiarities and subtle impressions on the axis of transfer and countertransference in the first stage to ascertain the existence of the past and how it haunts the present. In the second stage, these data are processed so that, in the third level, they are demonstrated to the analysand.

The intersubjective psychoanalyst Benjamin, wanting to present a metaphor of the interaction of the two psychic apparatuses, borrows an image from neuroscience: "The alarm bell of the patient's amygdala will ring in my ears, and then I will feel helpless in my analytic work." In a psychodynamic way, the above would become:

> I know that if the other is in a state of excessive stimulation, therefore in a traumatic mental condition – whether he feels excessive anxiety, excessive fear, or excessive shame – this means that I will not be able to listen to him because the intensity and weight of what he feels will

hinder me due to excessive quantity. The danger is that the analysand will very quickly leave this intolerable message. I will follow him on this flight if the observer inside me does not perceive the resulting disconnection, however light it may be. Then [the observer] he will turn attention to what was heard, and, above all, what was not heard just before the dysphonia.

(Benjamin 2007, 56)

The above psychoanalysts agree that a process of symbolization and crea-tion of representations of the heavy losses that have already taken place must first occur so that the lethargic aspects of the psychic apparatus can return to life (Scarfone 2011). For the sake of brevity and in this chap-ter's context, I will name the "past that does not pass away," calling it an "agalma." I borrow from the everyday Greek language a word that refers, on the one hand, to something immovable and frozen (therefore mentally dead and terrifying) and, on the other hand, to something that is a personal creation of the subject, and which is exposed to others (therefore, poten-tially, seductive). The agalma, meaning statue in the Greek language, is used as a metaphor for the state of part of the psyche that has lost the human identity and, therefore, the ability to speak and introspect. Analytical work aims to create space and time that will allow the agalma to come to life in these conditions.

Maria's case allows us to better look into the future of a grandchild of a refugee. In the case of refugees, we are often confronted with men who similarly leave their families because it is easier for them to migrate ille-gally and work in EU countries on their own. Maria's grandfather, about whom I will write below, abandoned his wife and 4-year-old son when a woman, an older, wealthy, and educated Latina, fell in love with him and proposed to take him with her to Latin America, where she promised to make him a prosperous factory owner. His decision to follow her was part of a more general social context in Greece at the time, where immigration was a frequent and forced solution for families who could not make ends meet. Often, the emigrated man started a new family abroad abandoning the one in Greece or sending them money. Sometimes, the man would take his wife with him, leaving the children with relatives who stayed behind to raise them.

Maria's grandfather became a wealthy entrepreneur with the help of the woman as promised, and he had 19 children with 19 different women to whom he sent money, as well as to the *mother and son* (the "couple") he had left behind. Could anyone have suspected in this frantic race in his per-sonal life that something was happening to him? Before migration, he was a faithful husband and father. How was he transformed?

In Ovid's *Metamorphoses*, where the myths of Greek and Roman antiq-uity are gathered, the metamorphosis comes either as a result of the subject's own will (for example, Daphne, chased by Apollo, begged her mother, Gaia, to help her transform into a tree when Apollo tried to rape her) or as punishment imposed by someone outside the subject (for example, Actaeon, who, unwittingly seeing Artemis naked bathing in a spring, was transformed by her into a deer and devoured by his dogs). Myths, literary works, and art in general can help people – and therefore caregivers and refugees – to endure the agony that is entwined with their lives, the ineffable suffering, and the cry of the suffering subject.

The refugee route is often placed at the crossroads of collective trauma and individual choice or fate. Psychoanalysis, with its attention to agitation due to the trauma of past internalized relationships with the object and deepening of the defensive processes that any loss mobilizes, can offer the refugee caregiver a view of the potential intergenerational destiny of the trauma and reinforce his desire to intervene as quickly as possible.

Clinical Material

Maria, a 16-year-old teenager, suddenly began to say "crazy things" that worried her mother. For example, she suddenly "realized" that she had been hit by a truck and had died. She refused to leave the house.

At our first meeting I saw a teenager who was scared but also cute, with a modern hairstyle that revealed coquetry and made me optimistic about the outcome of the therapeutic relationship we would develop.

It quickly became apparent that her father was the dominant relationship in her life. The two have lived in a closed system since Maria was born. Through relevant questions, however, I concluded that Maria was neither now nor before in a psychotic disorder. Her ego remained unfragmented and she was able to maintain its perceptual ability of the reality. Maria probably belonged to the hysterical structures where the danger of fragmentation permanently threatens the psyche, but without the ego losing the ability to successfully defend itself.

Maria experienced the mother as absent and indifferent. She worked a lot and slept when she was at home. The father had no substantial relationship with the mother. He was constantly occupied with Maria, whom he admired immensely.

He considered her capable of becoming important in any field she pursued, from a great writer (when Maria won an award at school for writing an essay on the importance of savings) to a violin soloist (when the teacher at the conservatory praised her progress). As a result, Maria abandoned all activities under the weight of the demands of her father's fantasies. However, she could not feel the slightest anger against him or think that there was anything morbid about it.

The intelligent and sensitive father had been welcomed by his [then future] wife's family when he was left around 16, alone in the neighborhood, after his mother's second marriage. In the first period of Maria's treatment, there was no mention of her paternal grandfather, and no thought of intergenerational trauma occurred to me. The incestuous fantasies of a daughter fixated on the Oedipus phase because of a father's long preoccupation with her and a devaluation of the mother at home were not enough. It was obvious that Maria's mother could not claim her daughter from the father, who was mentally breaking down every time Maria moved away and focused entirely on her work and life outside the home.

Despite her fear of me, Maria gradually began to tell me about her peers' groups, complaining that they did not include her in their meetings. Everything seemed to happen in accordance with her age, except for the intensity of a sudden erotic daze that seized her a year and a half later and that easily transferred from one of the boys her age to a second one when the first did not reciprocate. With this second young man, Maria entered into an intense relationship, as traumatic as the one with her father. The young man was pathologically jealous of her and would not let her move away from him. Maria did not react to it because it felt familiar, accepting the repetition of the pattern as if it were a natural phenomenon.

Relieved by Maria's removal from the relationship with the father and at the same time worried about the massive investment in the young man, I had an indeterminate sense of danger. One of Maria's dreams from this period illustrated the "closing of the door" that we faced a little later.

Maria's dream: Maria is at home. Someone knocks on the door. Maria looks through the peephole of the door and then realizes that someone else is in the room lying down and sleeping. She feels she has to protect him and does not open the door.

Her associations: Maria says her father avoids opening the door or answering the phones because people are stalking him – he owes money to many.

I think that Maria realizes that someone is asleep when there is a knock on her door and tries to "see" through the peephole. Is this the same person who is both outside and inside? Stranger and yet so familiar! What other interpretation could I think of?

After a few evenings, in a dream of mine I saw that they imposed on me and another a joint task. He suddenly fell asleep, and while at first I felt abandoned, I thought that in this way he gives me the opportunity to refuse to do what has been imposed on us.

My associations: The sudden sleep of my partner reminded me of when I woke up to Maria's dream. I thought it was perhaps a "twin dream" of what I am used to paying attention to. According to the theory of the Swiss psychoanalyst Benedetti, a twin dream is a "transitional subject." I thought that in my countertransference I felt helpless, and, in search of a father, I turned to Benedetti.

My dream, of course, was present in my mind when, after a few weeks, Maria left a message on voicemail saying that she should stop her analysis because she just realized that she was pregnant, and the gynecologist told her that it would be dangerous to terminate the pregnancy. The pregnancy was advanced, and Maria did not realize it.

I suggested that she come one last time. She accepted with obvious reluctance. She was scared because she was sure I would insist that she continue her therapy.

Having in mind the above twin dreams, hers and mine, I reminded her of her dream and I told her that the pregnancy seemed to be an escape from an unwanted, persecuting person. On the other hand, I told her that things won't be as easy for her in the coming years. I added that she can return to therapy if and when she feels like it.

She returned after five years because, as she said, I was the only one who, at that moment, did not advise her in a simplistic way: Yes or No.

After a difficult pregnancy, her parents were divorced, her father was homeless and sick, her mother returned to her mother, and she now lived in a village. She did not work and lived with the help of an aunt. The father of her child neither abandoned her nor was he close to her in any way, holding her "hostage." The situation looked worse than I had predicted.

At that time, looking for the good decision about Maria's therapy (Maria had no money at that time to pay for the sessions) and wondering about the debt of the dream, I presented this case to colleagues. I was surprised to hear one of them say that this is a classic, incestuous relationship between a father and a hysterical daughter that culminates in a happy gestation and the advent of new life in the world.

I decided that I would take her on but she would pay me a small, symbolic, amount for a short period (maximum six months) until she found work.

With my help, Maria studied cooking, found a job and distanced herself from her son's father, and gradually became reacquainted with her father's story. As I have already written, her father's father had followed a wealthy woman in Latin America and had 19 other children by 19 different women. Her father stayed with his mother who, somehow, was stunned "as if she had been hit by a truck," for many years. Her life ended there, as she had been saying for years. When her son met his father, at the latter's invitation to the hospital bed where he would die, did the mother feel free? Betrayed? Either way, the mother formed a relationship with someone who physically abused her, and her son decided to live alone, at the age of 16. Then he was "adopted" by Maria's mother's family.

History repeats itself: a father who leaves, a relationship of attachment between mother and child, a life on the fringes of society outside the usual social networks of relationships.

I accompanied Maria to this part of her life where she struggled to find work to raise her child and herself and where she was gradually able to make friendly relationships with girls of the same age – at first, they also took on an erotic connotation whose transferential side did not escape her. The relationships with men that followed were reprints of the relationship with her father.

Gradually, we find the words for the memory of the disaster in her father's life. Maria decides to take her 14-year-old son with her and emigrate abroad – to Europe and not to Latin America. Does she follow her grandfather? Does she realize her father's unformed dream of following his father with his mother abroad? The teenage son settles in well and shows excellent progress in school and relationships, while she tries to be able to say "no" to derogatory behavior from employers and partners.

Elements of Theory

Maria did not have a good grasp of reality. It was not just that she feared she had been hit by a truck and had died. These thoughts subsided relatively quickly, although the sensitivity of a hypochondriac nature has remained to this day. However, it seemed that it was not clear to her what it meant to get pregnant and have a child whose father barely recognized it. Or what it meant for her to remain without a professional identity and no income.

At the same time, her incomplete perception of reality was accompanied by several good mental and psychic abilities that seemed to support her father's grandiose fantasies, which partly affected her as well. However, instead of helping her to form a core of healthy ambition, for many years, these fantasies immobilized her in order to avoid either a maniac pursuit of their realization or a painful experience of defeat.

The identification with her father was conscious from the beginning. According to Maria, he was intelligent and, at the same time, very different from others and isolated. He adored his daughter. He had no reason to stay with the family after she had a child – it was her escape from the incestuous father and not the child they had together. Maria's father felt abandoned once more and left the house.

The quest for a father is central to one's life – the whole Odyssey begins with the search for Odysseus by Telemachus, who travels to find his father. Volkan in his book *Migrants and Refugees* (2017) refers to his work with members of the American World War II Orphans Network (2014). ;In interviews with many of these children (when they were 50–60 years old) whose father had died in the war, often before they were born or when they were very young, he discovered that they had created completely imaginary depictions of the father with the help of photographs and narratives from their mother or other members of the family.

In other words, while they had no conscious memories of the lost parent, later, through the photographs and stories they heard about their [to them] unknown father, they created partially, or in a more comprehensive way, little by little, and with the help of the people close to them, representations of their father, which however were fantasies. The above representations, constructed naturally according to their needs, desires, and fears, contributed significantly to the processes of identity creation but simultaneously proved to be very rigid, grandiose, and mysterious. A great pride mostly accompanied them because their father had lost his life during the war. However, as a result of this process, they had equally grandiose representations that forced them to constantly affirm their difference from their peers, creating a condition of loneliness and false self.

I think that the mixture of betrayal and pride is often found in children who "lost" their father when he immigrates for any reason. This mixture can be transmitted in their own children, asking them to be constantly with them and to make them proud. Maria's father asked her to be always with him and to mirror him as an exceptional person.

I will mention the work of G. Benedetti, whose thinking about psychoses and psychotic nuclei has influenced my practice described above. I have found the concept of the *transitional subject* remarkably manageable and, in particular, its appearance in the form of twin dreams (Benedetti 1995, 1998).

More specifically, Benedetti argues that, in psychodynamic-type therapies of psychotic patients, parts of the analysand's mind enter the analyst's inner psychic life when the latter does not resort defensively to hasty intellectualizations and interpretations. Benedetti coined the term transitional subject to speak of something that can be a visual projection of the analyst, a work of art, a dream or fantasy of the analyst, and, generally, a form that unites the analysand and analyst. One such creation of the therapist's unconscious is a twin dream, i.e., a dream that continues the theme of the patient's dream and changes it from within. The advent of the transitional subject in the analyst's consciousness is often a surprise to him, potentially a revelation of meaning (Benedetti 1995).

A concept analogous to the transitional subject is Ogden's best-known term of the analytical third (1994). In attempting to capture the intersubjective quality of the analytical relationship, Ogden introduced the *analytic third*, which is a creation of the analyst and the analysand which, in turn, are creations of the third subject of the analysis. In this conception of the analytical process, the experience must be coconstructed in interaction with someone else, in this case, with the analyst.

The moment of interruption of Maria's first period of therapy, amid excessive, manic stimulation, is potentially a sign of a return to the present of a "past that does not pass away"; in other words, of a past that has not yet been formulated into a mnemonic trace. The exit from time and the collapse of the social bond are accompanied by the classic defenses investigated in disasters:

(1) *Denial:* Nothing significant has happened. (2) *Identification with the aggressor:* Maria was not even taking contraception. (3) *The survivor's guilt:* Why would she live when her parents had "died" mentally? Why live leading a fetus to its death? (4) *The distortion of judgment:* The young man will become a good father, and if this is not done, then Maria's father can raise the new child as his own.

The above defenses signal, for analysts who have dealt with trauma, the entry into "war." Once the area of trauma is perceived, war comes to transference, and perhaps not metaphorically. Then, it is necessary to traverse the landscape of destruction with the analyst not having the correct interpretation, anxious to find it but having to work on his cracks in a temporality out of time, in an attempt to construct a memory that can be forgotten.

The rupture points of this flow create within the analysis points of rupture of the synchronization between the analyst and the analysand, the value of the recognition of which is emphasized. At the same time, the experience of betrayal becomes an important issue through the therapeutic relationship, and the analyst must work in such a way as to restore the experience of a world that operates under specific laws. In *Talks on Psychanalysis*, J. Benjamin uses the concept of the moral third to illustrate the above function of the third term – beyond and in addition to the symbolic third term of the analytical process (Benjamin 2018).

Reparation in cases of extreme trauma takes place only through acknowledging the trauma and suffering that it entails. Acknowledgment involves confirmation of receipt, acceptance that something happened. Telling Maria that she escapes but she "sleeps," denying the difficulty of her decision, I acknowledged the traumatic situation of a father's escape from poverty, leaving a moral debt toward the son left behind. Moreover, I accepted being "betrayed" and left behind without ceasing to feel and think about the one who left, here Maria. I insisted on caring for her.

Bibliography

Akhtar, S. (1995). A third individuation: Immigration, Identity, and the Psychoanalytic process. *Journal of the American Psychoanalytic Association* 43: 1051–1084.

Benedetti, G. 1995. *La mort dans l'âme*. Translated by P. Faugeras. Ramonville-Sainte-Agne, Paris: Erès.

Benedetti, G. 1998. *Le sujet emprunté*. Translated by P. Faugeras. Ramonville-Sainte-Agne, Paris: Erès.

Benjamin, J. 2007. "Listening Together: Intersubjective Aspects of the Analytic Process of Losing and Restoring Recognition." In *Listening to Others: Developmental and Clinical Aspects of Empathy and Attunement*, edited by Salman Akhtar, 53–77. London: Jason Aronson.

Benjamin, J. 2018. "How Therapy With Victims of Political Trauma Repairs the Third: Commentary on Gómez and Kovalskys's Work in the Context of post dictatorship Chile." *Psychoanalytic Dialogues* 28: 115–21.

Bion, W. 1962. *Learning from Experience. In Seven Servants (1977)*. New York: Aronson.

Brenner, I. (2002). "On survival and remembrance." *Journal of Applied Psychoanalytic studies* 4: 3–11.

Breuer, J., and S. Freud. 1895. *Studies on Hysteria*. S.E. 2: 1–323.

Damasio, A. 1999. *Le sentiment même de soi*. Translated by C. Larsonneur and C. Tiercelin. Paris: Odile Jacob.

Davoine, F., and J.-M. Gaudilliere. 2004. *Histoire et Trauma. In Greek. History and Trauma (2013)*. Translated by Marina Kounezis. Curated by Yiannis Gkiastas. Athens: Methexis Publications.

DeM'Uzan, M. 1970. "Le même et l'identique." *Revue française de psychanalyse* 34: 441–51.

DeM'Uzan, M. 1993. "Interprétation et Mémoire." *Revue française de psychanalyse* 57 (1): 7–20.

DeM'Uzan, M. 2013. *Death and Identity: Being and the Psycho-Sexual Drama*. London and New York: Routledge.

Eilenberger, W. 2018. *The Age of the Magi: The Great Ten Years of Philosophy 1919–1929*. Translated by Koilis Giannis. Athens: Patakis Publications.

Erikson, E. H. 1956. "The Problem of Ego Identity." *Journal of the American Psychoanalytic Association* 4: 56–121.

Erikson, E. H. 1964. "Identity and Uprootedness in Our Time." In *Insight and Responsibility*, edited by Erik H. Erikson, 81–107. New York: Norton.

Freud, S. 1911. "Psychoanalytic Notes on an Autobiographical Account of a Case of Paranoia (Dementia Paranoides)." *S.E.* 12: 1–82.

Freud, S. 1915. "The Unconscious." *S.E.* 14: 159–215.

Freud, S. 1923. "The Ego and the Id." *S.E.* 19: 1–66.

Freud, S. 1932. "New Introductory Lectures XXXI: The Dissection of the Psychical Personality." *S.E.* 22: 57–80.

Giannoulaki, C. 2020. *Heinz Kohut: Narcissism and Psychoanalysis*. Athens: Indiktos.

Giannoulaki, C. 2023. "Is Psychoanalysis of Any Help for Refugees?" In *Trauma, Flight and Migration: Psychoanalytic Perspectives*, edited by the series IPA in the Community. London and New York: Routledge.

Hartokollis, 1972. "Time as a Dimension of Affects." *Journal of the American Psychoanalytic Association* 20: 92–108.

Hartokollis, P. 1983. *Time and Timelessness: The Varieties of Temporal Experience—A Psychoanalytic Inquiry*. New York: International Universities Press.

Hartokollis, P. 2006. *Time and Timelessness: Variations of Temporal Experience (A Psychoanalytic Approach)*. Athens: Kastaniotis.

Jacobs, T. 1986. "On Countertransference Enactments." *Journal of the American Psychoanalytic Association* 34: 289–307.

Jacobson, E. 1964. *The Self and the Object World*. New York: International Universities Press.

Kafka, F. 1915. *Metamorphosis. Greek Edition: Metamorphosis (2012)*. Translated by Margarita Zachariadou. Athens: Patakis Publications.

Kernberg, O. (2008). The Destruction of Time in Pathological Narcissism. *International Journal of Psychoanalysis* 89 (2): 299–312.

Kestenberg, J. S. (1980). Psychoanalyses of children of survivors from the Holocaust: Case presentations and assessment. *Journal of the American Psychoanalytic Association* 28 (4): 775–804.

Kestenberg, J. and Brenner, I. (1996). *The last witness: The child survivor of the Holocaust*. Washington, DC: American psychiatric Press.

Kestenberg, J. and Kahn, C. (1998). *Children surviving persecution*. Westport, CT: Greenwood.

Kogan, I (2002a). "Enactment" in the lives and treatment of Holocaust survivors' offspring. *Psychoanalytic Quarterly* 71: 251–272.

Kogan , I. (2002b). International handbook of multigenerational legacies of trauma. By Yael Danieli, New York: Plenum Publishing Corporation, 1998. *Journal of Applied Psychoanalytic Studies* 4: 93–97.

Kogan, I. (2019). Holocaust studies and the nature of evidence.: Commentaries on Gomolin's "The intergenerational transmission of Holocaust trauma: A psychoanalytic theory revisited" *Psychoanalytic Quarterly* 88: 525–540.

Lafarge, L. 2014. "On Time and Deepening in Psychoanalysis." *Psychoanalytic Dialogues* 24: 304–316.

Levine, H. B. 2009. "Time and Timelessness: Inscription and Representation." *Journal of the American Psychoanalytic Association* 57: 333–55.

Lifton, R. J. 1968. *Death in Life: Survivors of Hiroshima*. New York: Random House.

Lifton, R. J. 1972. "On Psychohistory." *Psychoanalysis and Contemporary Science* 1: 355–72.

Lifton, R. J. 1973. "The Sense of Immortality: On Death and the Continuity of Life." *American Journal of Psychoanalysis* 33 (1): 3–15.

Lifton, R. J. 1976. "From Analysis to Formation: Towards a Shift in Psychological Paradigm." *Journal of the American Academy of Psychoanalysis* 4: 63–94.

Masson, J. M. (1985). *The complete letters of Sigmund Freud to Wilhelm Fliess, 1887–1904*. London: Harvard University Press.

Niederland, W. G. 1968. "Clinical Observations on the Survivor Syndrome." *International Journal of Psychoanalysis* 75: 3–19.

Niederland, W. G. 1981. "The Survivor Syndrome: Further Observations and Dimensions." *Journal of the American Psychoanalytic Association* 29 (2): 413–25.

Ovid. 1966. *Metamorphoses*. [The entire work has never been trans. into Greek.] Selection of passages by Theodoros Yannatos. Athens: Difros.

Ogden, T. H. 1990. *The Matrix of the Mind: Object Relations and the Psychoanalytic Dialogue*. Northvale and London: Jason Aronson.

Ogden, T. H. 1994. "The Analytic Third: Working with Intersubjective Clinical Facts." *International Journal of Psychoanalysis* 49 (2): 313–15.

Ogden, T. H. 2004. "This Art of Psychoanalysis: Dreaming Undreamt Dreams and Interrupted Cries." *International Journal of Psychoanalysis* 85: 857–77. In Greek (2023). Translated by E. Kanellopoulou, I. Malogiannis, and M. Tzinieri Kokkosi. Athens: Icarus.

Papadopoulos, R. K. (2002). "Refugees, home and trauma." In *Therapeutic care for refugees: No place like home*, edited by R.K. Papadopoulos, 9–39. London: Karnac.

Papadopoulos, R. K. (2007). Refugees, trauma, and adversity-activated development. *European Journal of Psychotherapy and Counselling*, 9(3): 301–312.

Pelegrinis, N. T. 2009. *Dictionary of Philosophy*. Athens: Ellinika Grammata.

Purtill, C. 2021. "It's Time to Talk About Survivor's Guilt." *New York Times*, July 20.

Ricoeur, P. 1986. *Le mal: Un défi à la philosophie et la théologie*. In Greek (2006). Translated by Giorgos Grigoriou. Athens: Polis.

Sang-Hun, C. 2023. "Haunted by Guilt, Vilified Online: A Year After the Seoul Crowd Crash." *New York Times*, October 23.

Scarfone, D. 2006. "A Matter of Time: Actual Time and the Production of the Past." *Psychoanalytic Quarterly* 75: 807–34.

Scarfone, D. (2011). Repetition: Between presence and meaning. *Canadian Journal of Psychoanalysis* 19: 70–86.

Van Der Kolk, B. A., A. C. McFarlane, and L. Weisaeth. 1996. *Traumatic Stress*. New York: Guilford Press.

Varvin, S (2013). Trauma as non-verbal communication. Zeitschrift fur psychoanalytische theorie und praxis. 28(1): 114–130.

Volkan, V. D. (2014). "Father quest and linking objects: A story of the American World War II Orphans Network (AWON) and Palestinian orphans." In *Healing in the wake of parental loss: Clinical applications and therapeutic strategies*, edited by P. Cohen, M. Sossin & R. Ruth, 283–300. New York: Jason Aronson.

Volkan, V. D. (2017). *Immigrants and Refugees. Trauma, Perennial Mourning, Prejudice and Border Psychology*. Great Britain: Karnac.

Conclusion

Extreme aggression was recognized by Freud, especially after World War I, when, for example, he argued the following position:

> Men are not gentle creatures who want to be loved, and who at the most can defend themselves if they are attacked. On the contrary, they are creatures whose instinctual endowments are to be reckoned with a powerful share of aggressiveness. Who, in the face of all his life and history experience, will have the courage to dispute this assertion?
>
> (Freud 1930, 67)

Many, for example, the professor of Philosophy and award-winning author David Livingstone Smith (2011), believe that humans possess an inherent tendency to dehumanize, demean, and even kill. The easiest way to kill others is by divesting them of their individual humanity (Knafo and Lo Bosco 2017, 17).

The refugees flee violence, wars, poverty, political persecution, torture, and other catastrophes and flee evil in its multiple forms. Refugees as a group experience the most prolonged and extreme dehumanization today. Psychoanalysis, and even more, this book, does not propose a "solution" to the "problem" of refugees.

Work with Refugees

However, as psychoanalysts, we have some tools to explore the human mind in depth. Every day, we do research work to listen to the others – their unconscious and their "ghosts" included. In our everyday practice, we are concerned with the individual trying to listen not only to the unconscious, meaning to what is dissociated and split off, but also to what is still unrepresented and unable to be thought. We do the previous work through the psychoanalyst's conscious, preconscious, and unconscious experiences during the initial individual consultation and later individual and group psychotherapies (Christopoulous et al. 2023).

Psychoanalysis has a broad and humanistic character in rehumanizing the individual by facilitating the connection process to others and

DOI: 10.4324/9781003639022-14

helping to reestablish essential human bonds (Varvin 2019). The question is whether psychoanalysis can utilize its knowledge to improve the treatment of people outside the analytic setting.

Nowadays, the concept of the analytic setting has changed (Lemma 2017). The analytic setting is considered a structure in the analyst's mind, "a psychic arena in which such concepts define reality as symbolism, fantasy, transference, and unconscious meaning" (Parsons 2007, 1444). So, we can estimate the only encounter of a psychoanalyst with a refugee to be a psychoanalytic one. The point of interest is put on the internal work done in the psychoanalyst's mind to offer an exit from the inhuman traumatic experience to both the analyst and the refugee.

Moreover, psychoanalysis has a rich representational vocabulary. So, helped by this vocabulary, psychoanalysts can try to resist evil and try to represent it. Traumatized people suffer mental and bodily pains that are challenging to understand and difficult to put into words. Psychoanalysts have the tools to face the deficiencies in the representational system related to traumatic experiences. Understandably, there is increasing evidence that psychoanalytic therapies are helpful for traumatized people in comprehensive ways. Psychodynamic psychotherapy for traumatized patients is found to result in continued improvement after treatment ends (Schottenbauer 2008).

Work with Carers

Psychoanalysis can encourage people who work with refugees to turn their attention to their inner world and to face the "difficult" emotions that are evoked by getting close to the "inhuman" violence.

On the one hand, psychoanalytically oriented supervision aims to facilitate movement toward the other, initially turning toward introspection, the understanding of our own experience.

On the other hand, there can be no empathy from people (carers) who experience an unfair and inhumane attitude toward themselves. So, support and supervision for the carers of the refugees is of great help.

Work with the Community

Also, more involvement is needed with residents, who often feel that refugees are better cared for than they are. It is thus possible to avoid the polarization that follows the meeting with Xenos. In an environment of insecurity and collective anxiety, refugees may represent Xenos. Xenos in ancient Greek means the Other, the outsider, the visitor, the wanderer. Moreover, Xenos is also sacred. The intense xenophobia with which we react to refugees has its source in fear of the "Xenos." Ambivalence toward the stranger caught Freud's attention, particularly in the text Das Unheimlich (1919). Ambivalence toward refugees is one of the main characteristics of the affects in the caring person and/or the group, thus a trait of countertransference in the psychoanalytic glossary.

Work with Candidates of Psychoanalytical Societies and Psychoanalysts: Psychosis and Trauma Revisited

Last but not least, this book aims to remind the clinical usefulness not to forget the "psychotic patient" and his transference. The psychoanalytic theories on the treatment of psychotic patients are of great help when the analysand's self collapses for any reason. I particularly referred to the psychoanalyst Gaetano Benedetti (1998, 2002) and his thinking on the technique to turn the negative psychotic experience into a positive one through the construction of the "transitional subject."

"Paradoxically, research with psychotics reveals cognitive issues, connected with sociohistorical realities and the attendant emotions, that are accessible only via the transference" (Davoine and Gaudilliere 2004, 24–5). Refugees are not psychotic; on the contrary, they are often strong people who have survived many catastrophes. However, as Cohen (1985) wrote, we are often dealing with a psychotic experience anchored in reality events (p. 166) (in Boulanger 2007, 3). We believe that psychoanalytic theory may be equipped to address it, changing its technique and not interpreting and emphasizing the analytic understanding of transference and countertransference axis, as described in this book's clinical cases.

If people are ready for this overwhelming journey into the treatment of refugees, they can feel, hopefully, more "human" in the end. I quote Tina Packer, who declares that acting is not about putting on a character but discovering the character within you: you are the character; you just have to find it within yourself – albeit a significantly expanded version of yourself. Similarly, the analyst who treats refugees has to find a significantly expanded version of himself in order to connect with the "dead," disavowed, denied, and traumatized parts of the refugee. This is not about repression; this is about creating a link between human beings from a place haunted by "ghosts."

Psychosis and extreme trauma define a frontier of the human condition. If psychoanalysis wants to be of any help – and its tools are effective in enhancing the mentalization and the connection of the broken links – we have to adventure ourselves, exploring with the refugees new territories and acquiring new identities. The third individuation can apply to all of us, not only to refugees (Akhtar 1995).

To paraphrase Freud's simile of psychoanalysis as a small light in the much greater darkness of the unconscious, we might wonder whether psychoanalytic theory and clinical practice believe it is their task to illuminate with their small light, the darkness of unconscious forces, often destructive but also serving the construction of links, the Eros.

We come as strangers who are unable to communicate. At the same time we possess the spontaneous movement toward others and toward relating. The effort to meet and heal through human communication remains our weapon. Against the Evil we can construct a safe place to be together with, the humanistic values as a precious harbor.

Bibliography

Akhtar, Salman. 1995. "A Third Individuation: Immigration, Identity, and the Psychoanalytic Process." *Journal of the American Psychoanalytic Association* 43: 1051–84.

Benedetti, Gaetano. 1998. Le Sujet Emprunté: Le Vécu Psychotique du Patient et du Thérapeute. Paris: Éditions Érès, Coll. La Maison Jaune.

Benedetti, Gaetano. 2002. La Psychothérapie des Psychoses Comme Défi Existentiel. Paris: Éditions Érès, Coll. La Maison Jaune.

Boulanger, Ghislaine. 2007. *Wounded by Reality: Understanding and Treating Adult Onset Trauma.* New York and London: Psychology Press, Taylor & Francis Group.

Christopoulos, Anna, Giannoulaki, Chrysi, Tzavaras, Nicholas. 2023. "Mourning and Issues of Identity in the Treatment of Refugees in Lesvos." In *Trauma, Flight, and Migration: Psychoanalytic Perspectives,* edited by IPA in the Community, 119-31. London and New York: Routledge.

Cohen, J. (1985). Trauma and repression. *Psychoanalytic Inquiry.* 5: 161–90.

Davoine, Françoise, and Jean-Max Gaudillière. 2004. Histoire et Trauma. Trans. into Greek by Kounezis, Marina, curated by Gkiastas, Yiannis. 2013. Athens: Methexis.

Freud, S. 1919. The Uncanny SE 17: 217–56.

Freud, S. 1930. Civilization and its discontents. SE 21: 64–145.

Knafo, D. and Lo Bosco. (2017). *The age of perversion. Desire and Technology in Psychoanalysis and Culture.* London and New York: Routledge.

Lemma, Alessandra. 2017. *The Digital Age on the Couch: Psychoanalytic Practice and New Media.* London and New York: Routledge.

Livingstone Smith, David. 2011. *Less than Human: Why We Demean, Enslave, and Exterminate Others.* New York: St. Martin's Press.

Livingstone Smith, David. 2020. *On Inhumanity: Dehumanization and How to Resist It.* London: Oxford University Press.

Parsons, Michael. 2007. "Raiding the Inarticulate: The Internal Analytic Setting and Listening Beyond Countertransference." *International Journal of Psychoanalysis* 88: 1441–56.

Ricoeur, Paul. 1967. *The Symbolism of Evil.* Translated by Emerson Buchanan. New York: Harper & Row.

Ricoeur, Paul. 1986. *Le Mal: Un Défi à la Philosophie et à la Théologie.* Trans. Grigoriou, Giorgos. Athens: Patakis Publications.

Schottenbauer, Michele A., Carol R. Glass, Diane B. Arnkoff, and Sarah H. Gray. 2008. "Contributions of Psychodynamic Approaches to Treatment of PTSD and Trauma: A Review of the Empirical Treatment and Psychopathology Literature." *Psychiatry: Interpersonal and Biological Processes* 71 (1): 13–34.

Varvin, Sverre. 2019. "Psychoanalysis and the Situation of Refugees: A Human Rights Perspective." In *Psychoanalysis, Law, and Society,* edited by Massimo Montagna and Susan Harris. London: Routledge/CRC Press on May 21, 2019. Available online: https://www.crcpress.com/Psychoanalysis-Law-and-Society/Montagna-Harris/p/book/9780367194505 or https://www.routledge.com/Psychoanalysis-Law-and-Society/Montagna-Harris/p/book/9780367194505

Index

For Product Safety Concerns and Information please contact our EU
representative GPSR@taylorandfrancis.com
Taylor & Francis Verlag GmbH, Kaufingerstraße 24, 80331 München, Germany

www.ingramcontent.com/pod-product-compliance
Lightning Source LLC
Chambersburg PA
CBHW050611280326
41932CB00016B/2993